Understa Pacemaker

or
Defibrillator

What Patients and Families Need to Know

David L. Hayes, MD, FACC, FHRS

Consultant, Division of Cardiovascular Diseases
Mayo Clinic, Rochester, Minnesota
Professor of Medicine
College of Medicine, Mayo Clinic

Rebecca S. Fallon, MS

Certified Cardiac Device Specialist

Matthew D. Noble, BS

Certified Cardiac Device Specialist

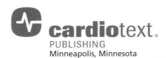

cardiotext.
PUBLISHING
Minneapolis, Minnesota

Cardiotext Publishing, LLC
3405 W. 44th Street
Minneapolis, Minnesota 55410
USA

www.cardiotextpublishing.com

Any updates to this book may be found at: www.cardiotextpublishing.com/titles/detail/9781935395553
Comments, inquiries, and requests for bulk sales can be directed to the publisher at: info@cardiotextpublishing.com.

This book is intended for educational purposes and to further general scientific and medical knowledge, research, and understanding of the conditions and associated treatments discussed herein. This book is not intended to serve as and should not be relied upon as recommending or promoting any specific diagnosis or method of treatment for a particular condition or a particular patient. It is the reader's responsibility to determine the proper steps for diagnosis and the proper course of treatment for any condition or patient, including suitable and appropriate tests, medications or medical devices to be used for or in conjunction with any diagnosis or treatment.

Due to ongoing research, discoveries, modifications to medicines, equipment and devices, and changes in government regulations, the information contained in this book may not reflect the latest standards, developments, guidelines, regulations, products, or devices in the field. Readers are responsible for keeping up to date with the latest developments and are urged to review the latest instructions and warnings for any medicine, equipment, or medical device. Readers should consult with a specialist or contact the vendor of any medicine or medical device where appropriate.

Except for the publisher's website associated with this work, the publisher is not affiliated with and does not sponsor or endorse any websites, organizations, or other sources of information referred to herein.

The publisher and the author specifically disclaim any damage, liability, or loss incurred, directly or indirectly, from the use or application of any of the contents of this book.

Unless otherwise stated, all figures and tables in this book are used courtesy of the authors.
Figures from Mayo Clinic are used by permission of Mayo Foundation for Medical Education and Research.
All rights reserved.

Library of Congress Control Number: 2012935734
ISBN: 978-1-935395-55-3

Printed in the United States of America.

www.cardiotextpublishing.com/titles/detail/9781935395553

This book is dedicated to the patients and families we have had the privilege to touch either directly or indirectly in our respective careers.

Table of Contents

Acknowledgments   vi

Preface   vii

Foreword   xi

Chapter 1. Normal and Abnormal Heart Function   1

Chapter 2. Types of Devices   17

Chapter 3. Before Your Device Procedure   27

Chapter 4. Inside the Procedure Room (Operating Room)   45

Chapter 5. What Next? After Your Procedure   53

Chapter 6. Follow-Up Care   65

Chapter 7. Possible Complications   77

Chapter 8. The Shocking Truth   93

Chapter 9. Living with a Device   105

Chapter 10. Other Important Issues   123

Appendix 1: Patient Resources Online   135

Appendix 2: Understanding Abbreviations for Devices   137

Glossary   141

Index   149

Acknowledgments

The authors acknowledge colleagues who assisted in critical review of this text:

- Jodie Alwin, MBA
- Monica Boege, RN
- Rosemary Horsman, RN
- Marjorie Martin, RN
- Brian Powell, MD
- Melissa Rott, RN
- Samuel F. Sears, PhD
- Wayne M. Sotile, PhD
- Tracy Webster, RN

Preface

I remember the first time I ever heard about the implantable defibrillator. There I was, a scared 17-year-old, too proud to admit my fears, lying in a hospital bed. I had just survived my fifth cardiac arrest. Having been fortunate enough to survive such an ordeal, my family and I were looking for answers.

My doctors soon explained that an ICD was my best treatment option, and within a few days, I underwent my first ICD implant. Over the course of the next 18 years, this device would literally save my life more than 20 times and deliver so many shocks that I would lose count. I would get shocked while sleeping, while awake, while passed out, and while conscious. I would come to feel as if I'd seen it all.

However, the ICD would also keep me alive long enough to complete a college education and work as a cardio-pulmonary technician and research assistant at the University of Michigan, before going to work for one of the world's largest ICD manufacturers. I was hired at age 23, the youngest field employee in company history, as a clinical expert specializing in pacemakers and ICDs—and I learned the ins and outs of these life-saving devices.

It was a terribly exciting job and an incredibly gratifying career as well. I had the opportunity to see these devices, just like the one that saved my life almost yearly, from the inside and out, as both a healthcare worker and a patient. I would go on to get promoted to a sales position, in which I was responsible for educating physicians on the benefits of our ICDs, while I maintained my clinical responsibilities. And throughout all of this, every day, I was first and foremost an ICD patient.

Talking with hundreds of ICD patients, seeing them when things were good and when things were bad, was both a blessing and a curse at times. When I was having a problem of my own, it was great to know exactly what was happening from a technical standpoint. Yet, at times, it could be terribly frightening, as the unusual case with complications would inevitably come to mind, causing undue fear whenever my own heart would race uncontrollably, a sign that the ICD may need to intervene.

It was also through these hundreds of interactions with ICD patients from ages 4 to 96 that I realized there wasn't much available to help us patients get through the tough times. Sometimes, it felt as if even those closest to us were unable to understand what we were going through. That, in part, is what led me to write my first book, *One Beat at a Time: Living with Sudden Cardiac Death*.

One Beat at a Time, my autobiography, tells the story of what it was like to live with the threat of sudden cardiac death constantly looming, and then the threat of a shock always lurking in the back of my mind once the ICD was placed. With complete openness, it describes all my fears, thoughts, and prayers through all of my struggles. Yet that book was about me; my hope is that this book is about *you.*

This book was first born in a chance meeting at Mayo Clinic in Rochester, MN. I had been invited to speak to a group of patients and clinicians after *One Beat at a Time* was released. It was the first time I had been there since flying the thousand-mile journey on a Medevac 25 years earlier, as a 5-year-old clinging to life. Although I didn't remember any of my first trip to the Mayo Clinic, it was a bit surreal going back. I wasn't supposed to make it

Preface

out of the Mayo Clinic alive, let alone be returning, speaking as an invited guest, years later. It was exciting.

As it turned out, I would also have the chance to meet Dr. David Hayes while on this trip. Dr. Hayes had written multiple textbooks for medical professionals on pacemakers and ICDs. It was during this meeting with him that he mentioned that he was thinking of writing a book on cardiac devices *for patients*. I had thought the same thing, and in fact had already written the first half of this very Preface. Needless to say, I was incredibly excited to get an email in the days following, asking if I would like to co-author this book with him.

The project languished a bit, and frankly just didn't really get going until about a year later, when Rebecca Fallon was brought on board through another chance meeting with Dr. Hayes.

Rebecca is a specialist in ICD patient psychology. She obtained this specialty while working on her Masters of Science in clinical and health psychology at the University of Florida. She uses her degree daily while working in the medical education group of one of the manufacturers of implantable cardiac devices. She, like I, also spent several years working as a clinical expert for another major device manufacturer. Rebecca possesses a wealth of information on the psychology of patients with cardiac devices. More importantly, however, she brings experiences and education that neither Dr. Hayes nor I can offer.

Hopefully, the three of us have combined our expertise and experiences to offer you a medically solid, emotionally healthy, personal account of what your life with your device will be like. In fact, I expect that this book will answer most of the questions you may have about your device, or the device implanted in a loved one, and even answer questions you didn't know to ask. It is our most sincere hope that this book will provide you with the knowledge you need to live each day, thankful for this incredible, life-saving device.

This book will function as a technical manual. Should you have a specific question, go to the Index. For instance, looking up "battery" will direct you to the points in the book that speak of the battery life on your devices, giving you a clue as to what to expect. We also hope to address more than the technical here.

So whether you've just been told you need a cardiac device, or you've had one for years, we trust you'll find some hope, some information, and some peace of mind in the pages of this book.

—Matt Noble, March 2012

Foreword

Implantable cardiac devices—that is, pacemakers, implantable cardioverter defibrillators (ICDs), and cardiac resynchronization therapy (CRT) devices—are highly sophisticated electronic devices that are commonly used. In a perfect world, decision making regarding the use of these therapies would include a complete discussion of the pros and cons of treatment and ample time for questions and discussions with one's family and other healthcare providers. In real life, the recommendation for such a device often arises suddenly, and patients and family members may not have adequate time to get up to speed or even to begin to formulate questions to ask the caregivers involved.

The need for better information for patients and their families is critical. Valuable educational information can be difficult to find, and perhaps more difficult to comprehend and implement. Professional societies, patient advocacy groups, device manufacturers, and others have developed some excellent tools and educational materials about the devices themselves, the procedures required to place the devices, and follow-up care. However, the three of us writing this book felt that there was still a void. There was no single source that included all the information patients and their loved ones need and want.

As authors, we each bring different talents and experience to the effort, and we feel that the combination of our different backgrounds has resulted in a more complete source of information about receiving and living with an implantable cardiac device. From my perspective as a cardiologist, with my career largely focused on implantable cardiac devices, I have had the privilege of interacting with thousands of patients and their families as they confront healthcare decisions and learn to live with their devices. This has given me an opportunity to anticipate and appreciate the most common areas of confusion that arise when patients are told they need a cardiac device or during follow-up after its implantation. Matt Noble brings an important dual perspective as both a patient living with an implanted cardiac device and as a technical expert who previously held a position with a major cardiac device manufacturer. Matt describes his journey in the Preface, in a prior book,[1] and throughout this book. Rebecca Fallon also brings two unique attributes to this effort. She currently lives and breathes education related to implantable cardiac device therapy in her daily work with a major manufacturer. In addition, her formal training is in clinical and health psychology, and her understanding of health psychology informed our work by her additional insights to the fears and concerns that patients and families often face.

We hope that our combined professional and personal experiences have resulted in a meaningful and useful single source for anyone who may need or is currently living with an implantable cardiac device.

—David L. Hayes, MD

---

[1] *One Beat at a Time: Living with Sudden Cardiac Death.* 2005; Russell Douglas Publishing, 13097 Golfside Ct, Suite 103, Clio, MI, 48420.

Chapter I

Normal and Abnormal Heart Function

Learning more about the heart's normal structure and anatomy may help you understand why different heart problems occur and the conditions that may lead to the need for an implanted device.

BASIC CONCEPTS OF CARDIAC BLOOD FLOW

The heart is often described in terms of two concepts: "plumbing" and "electrical." The heart is, by definition, a pump. There are four chambers in the heart (Figure 1).

The two chambers on the top are the **atria** (singular: atrium), and the two bottom chambers are the **ventricles.** Although every part of the heart is important, the left ventricle is responsible for pumping blood throughout the body, and it therefore plays a vital role in blood circulation.

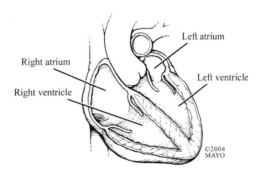

Figure 1. Normal heart.

When the left ventricle squeezes, the blood exits the heart through the **aortic valve** into a large blood vessel, the **aorta**. From there, the blood travels to all parts of the body (Figure 2). The blood leaving the left ventricle is rich with oxygen, which the rest of your body needs to stay healthy. As the blood goes through the aorta to other arteries and progressively smaller blood vessels, some of the oxygen in the blood leaves the red blood cells to nourish the body's tissues. The oxygen-poor blood then enters the **veins** and is routed back to the right side of the heart.

The blood enters the right atrium and then passes through a valve called the **tricuspid valve** into the right ventricle. When the right ventricle contracts or squeezes, the blood travels through the **pulmonic valve** into blood ves-

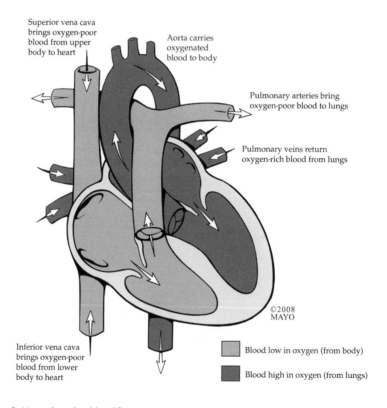

Figure 2. Normal cardiac blood flow.

sels in the lungs. In tiny vessels in the lungs, oxygen can pass back into the blood cells. Oxygen-rich blood then re-enters the left atrium (the top chamber on the left side of the heart) and goes through the **mitral valve** into the left ventricle, where the process starts all over again.

A very important term to be familiar with is the phrase left **ventricular ejection fraction,** abbreviated as LVEF or, sometimes, just EF. The LVEF is defined as the percentage or fraction of blood that the left ventricle squeezes out with each beat. Different hospitals and laboratories may use slightly different values for a "normal" LVEF. In general, a normal LVEF is 50 to 60% (See Figures 1 and 3). Some patients intuitively think that all the blood should be squeezed out, and that the LVEF should be 100%, but that would definitely *not* be normal or healthy. A desirable LVEF percentage is 50 to 60%.

The main function of the heart is to pump oxygen-rich blood throughout the body and then return the oxygen-poor blood to the lungs to regain oxygen.

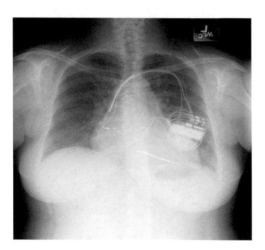

Figure 3. Figure 1 shows a diagram of the heart with normal ventricular size and normal wall thickness. With normal function the left ventricular ejection fraction should be 50% to 60%. By contrast, the chest x-ray featured in Figure 3 is from a patient with severe enlargement of the heart and the ejection fraction would be much below the normal limits.

However, the heart itself also needs blood supply. The **coronary arteries** supply the heart muscle with oxygen-rich blood. The coronary arteries come off the aorta, just above the heart valve from which blood exits the left ventricle (Figure 4). There is a right coronary artery and a left main coronary artery, which divides into two main branches: **the circumflex coronary artery** and the **left anterior descending coronary artery.** Although there can be many variations in the anatomy of the arteries, in general,

- the right coronary artery supplies the back wall (or **inferior** wall) of the left ventricle;

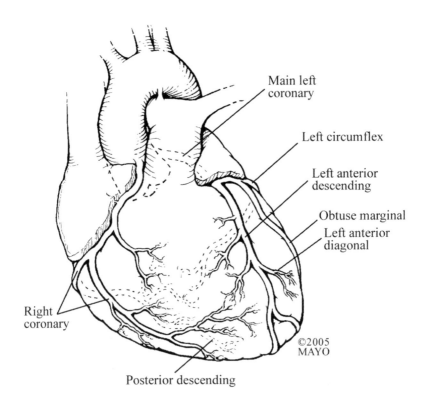

Coronary arteries carry blood to the heart muscle.
Dotted lines show arteries on the back of the heart.

Figure 4. Coronary arteries.

- the left anterior descending coronary artery comes down the front wall (or **anterior** wall) of the left ventricle and often supplies blood to the tip or apex of the left ventricle; and

- the circumflex coronary artery circles around to the outside (or **lateral** wall) of the left ventricle.

Each of these main arteries has a number of branches, some of which can be quite large. That's why you may hear of someone having bypass surgery that involved four or five arteries being bypassed. What this probably means is that all three main coronary arteries were bypassed, and in addition, one or more main-branch vessels were bypassed.

Bypass procedures are performed by a cardiovascular surgeon. However, if only one or two blood vessels have blockages, the common treatment is to open the blockage with a balloon and often also to place a **stent** in the artery to keep it open (Figure 5). These "interventional" procedures are usually performed by cardiologists, specifically, interventional cardiologists. They will sometimes be referred to as the "plumbers" because they open the "pipes" to get blood to the heart muscle.

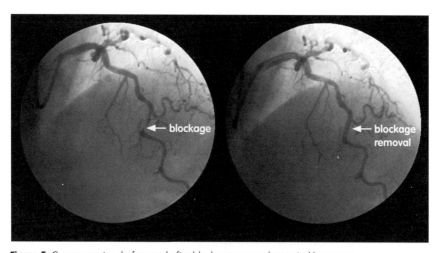

Figure 5. Coronary artery before and after blockage removal as noted by arrows.

The heart is able to pump because it is energized by its own electrical system. Remember the atria, right and left, are the top chambers of the heart. Located in the atria is very specialized tissue that forms the top "electrical switch." This is called the **sinus node,** and this is where the electrical impulse for the heart originates (Figure 6). When the sinus node "fires" or discharges, an electrical impulse is sent through both the right and left atria, resulting in the atria squeezing or "contracting." After traveling through the atria, the electrical impulse reaches more specialized tissue called the **atrioventricular (AV) node.** The AV node is a collection of cells located between the atria (A) and the ventricles (V), acting as somewhat of a relay switch. After passing through the AV node, the electrical impulse travels throughout the ventricles and results in ventricular squeezing, or contraction. More specifically, there are two main branches of electrical activation that come out of the AV node, called the **right bundle branch** and the **left bundle branch.** These branches carry the electrical impulse that results in ventricular activation.

Cardiologists who treat electrical problems of the heart are called **electrophysiologists** (*e-leck-tro-fizz-e-ol-o-gists*) or the "electricians" of the heart. If an implantable cardiac device is needed to help regulate the heart's electrical system, it is usually implanted by an electrophysiologist.

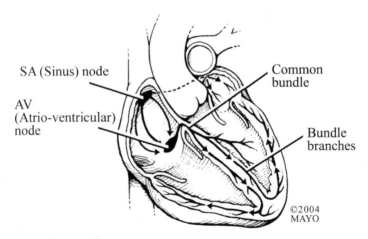

SA (Sinus) node

AV (Atrio-ventricular) node

Common bundle

Bundle branches

©2004 MAYO

Figure 6. Conduction pathways.

PROBLEMS WITH THE ELECTRICAL SYSTEM OF THE HEART

If you are reading this book, you, or someone close to you, may have an electrical problem with your (or their) heart. When you are talking to your caregivers, whether it is a nurse, technician, family doctor, cardiologist, electrophysiologist, or surgeon, a number of terms may be used that may be very confusing. (Throughout this book, we will usually refer to whoever is taking care of you or your loved one as the **caregiver**, realizing it can be one of many healthcare professionals.) You should feel comfortable taking this book with you when you talk to your caregivers, and if a term doesn't make sense or doesn't completely match up with the terms that are described below, speak up and ask them to clarify or explain what they mean.

Important Terms Explained

The terms **sinus node disease** and **sinus node dysfunction** are usually used interchangeably and simply mean there is a problem with the sinus node that was described above. Sinus node dysfunction may lead to slow heart rhythms (**bradycardias**) and/or fast heart rhythms (**tachycardias**). Sometimes the term **tachycardia-bradycardia syndrome** (or tachy-brady syndrome) may be used to describe sinus node dysfunction (Figure 7).

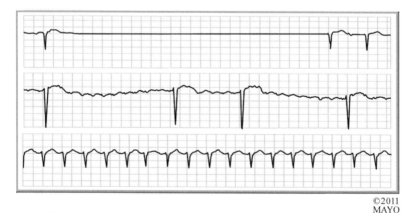

©2011
MAYO

Figure 7. Tachy-brady syndrome.

Sinus bradycardia simply means that the regular heart rate, determined by the sinus node, is slower than normal. What is "normal" depends on your age and your physical condition. An infant or small child normally has a faster heart rate than an adult. For an adult, a heart rate less than 60 beats per minute is technically considered sinus bradycardia. That is not to say, however, that all heart rates less than 60 beats per minute are a problem. Many adults, especially adults in good physical shape, may have resting heart rates in the 50s or even the 40s. In general, men have slower heart rates than women, and in general, our heart rates are slower at night when we are asleep. Slow heart rates usually do not require treatment unless they lead to symptoms, such as fatigue, lightheadedness, or decreased ability to do physical activity.

Sinus tachycardia means that the heart rate, as determined by the sinus node, is faster than normal. By definition, a tachycardia is a sinus rate greater than 100 beats per minute when you are at rest. Again, there will be variations. A rate of 100 in a very small child or infant may not be abnormal. If you are exercising or feverish, the heart rate will go up, and that's to be expected. Sinus tachycardia usually doesn't require treatment, although in some patients, a medication may be used.

Atrial fibrillation is a condition where there is irregular, rapid electrical activity in multiple areas of the atria. Atrial fibrillation may occur if the sinus node is abnormal and loses complete electrical control of the atria. During atrial fibrillation, the upper chambers of the heart are literally quivering (Figure 8). In this condition, there is absolutely no organized electrical activity of the upper chambers of the heart. Atrial fibrillation may lead to a very irregular beating of the ventricles because the atria are completely out of rhythm. If you experience atrial fibrillation, you may be aware of a fast and/or an irregular heartbeat.

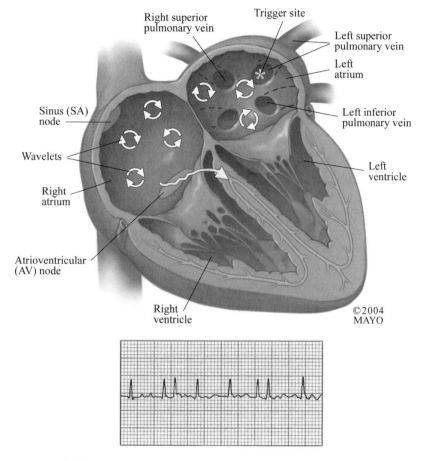

Figure 8. Atrial fibrillation.

Atrial flutter occurs when, instead of normal rhythm dictated by the sinus node, a more rapid and regular electrical activation of the top chambers of the heart results from continuous loop or pattern of electrical activity in the atria (Figure 9). Both atrial flutter and atrial fibrillation have the potential to result in your pulse going very fast, which may sometimes cause symptoms that need to be treated. Atrial flutter is a more organized electrical circuit in the atria, compared to atrial fibrillation.

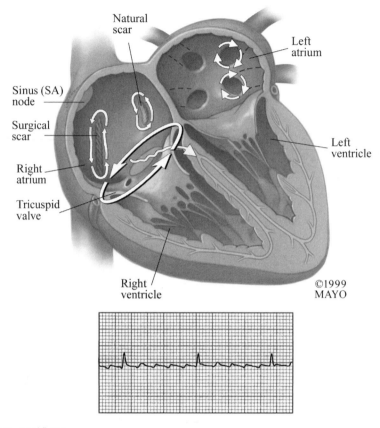

Natural scar

Left atrium

Sinus (SA) node

Surgical scar

Left ventricle

Right atrium

Tricuspid valve

Right ventricle

©1999 MAYO

Figure 9. Atrial flutter.

Heart block is a term you may hear your caregivers using, but it refers to an *electrical* block, and not a blockage in the arteries. To make it even more confusing, there can be several different types of heart block. Some types of heart block are problematic and require treatment, often with an implantable device, while other types of heart block are of no consequence and require no treatment. Therefore, it's worthwhile to explain the different types.

Types of Heart Block

First degree heart block refers to a very slight increase in the time it takes for an electrical impulse to leave your sinus node, electrify the atria, and get through the AV node. This delay is very short, literally thousandths of a second. Many people have a first degree heart block and, by itself, it is not concerning and does not require treatment.

Second degree heart block occurs when the electrical impulse is significantly delayed in getting through the AV node to the ventricles. Sometimes the delay is so long that the impulse does not make it through the AV node at all. This can result in "dropped" or "missed" heart beats since the ventricles do the majority of the pumping function of the heart. Patients with second degree heart block may miss only occasional heart beats, every other heart beat, or even several heart beats in a row (Figure 10). Depending on how many heart beats are being dropped, this condition could lead to a very slow heart rate and unpleasant symptoms, and may possibly require a pacemaker implant.

Third degree heart block means that there is a complete interruption of the electrical circuits through the AV node (Figure 11). This can lead to a very slow heart rate or no heart rate at all. Third degree heart block is usually

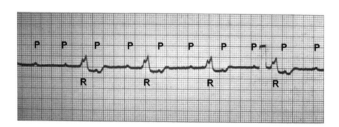

Figure 10. Tracing illustrating a second degree heart block—"P" indicates electrical activity from the atria or top chambers of the heart, and "R" indicates electrical activity from the ventricles or bottom chambers of the heart; there are two "P" waves for every single "R" wave.

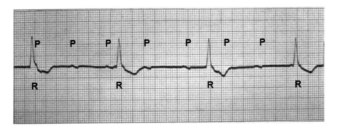

Figure 11. Tracing illustrating a third degree heart block—"P" indicates electrical activity from the atria or top chambers of the heart, and "R" indicates electrical activity from the ventricles or bottom chambers of the heart; there are more "P" waves than "R" waves, and there is no relationship between the "P's" and the "R's."

associated with severe symptoms such as passing out or, if left untreated, even death. A third degree heart block requires a pacemaker.

Left bundle branch block (LBBB) occurs when the electrical impulse is delayed getting through the left bundle branch of the electrical system in the ventricles. Some people will have LBBB with an otherwise normal heart, and may not have any specific problems or symptoms. In other people, a LBBB may be a sign that there has been damage to the heart muscle and resulting damage of an electrical pathway. It may also be a sign of a problem with the heart muscle that is unrelated to a heart attack (see below).

Right bundle branch block (RBBB), by contrast, means there is a delay through this specific electrical activating branch of the ventricles. RBBB is almost always a non-issue, meaning it is not associated with any specific heart problem and usually doesn't require any treatment.

There are other problems with the heart's electrical system that may be considered more serious because they originate in the ventricles, which are the two bottom chambers of the heart. These problems are covered in detail in Chapter 2.

Although these are the most common problems, there are other possible combinations of electrical problems in the heart. If your caregiver is telling you that you have some form of electrical blockage but it doesn't fit with the terms above, ask for more explanation.

PROBLEMS WITH THE BLOOD SUPPLY OF THE HEART

Damage to the systems that supply the heart with blood can lead to any of the electrical abnormalities described above, and may result in the need for an implanted device. Medically speaking, a heart attack or **myocardial infarction** is tissue death caused by a lack of blood flow—a "plumbing" problem. This is oftentimes confused with **sudden cardiac arrest,** an abnormal heart rhythm that causes loss of consciousness, which is actually an electrical issue. A heart attack—or more specifically, the damage caused by the lack of blood flow—can cause an episode of sudden cardiac arrest. This episode can follow within seconds of the heart attack, or may occur years later. Because of this, most people in the general public use the term "heart attack" to refer to both myocardial infarction and sudden cardiac arrest, not realizing that they are two very different issues, with very different treatments. Even so, sudden cardiac death is another example of an electrical issue that can be caused by a plumbing problem.

When a heart attack occurs, it typically involves a blockage of one of the coronary arteries. If the artery can be opened promptly, it may be possible to avoid any permanent damage to the heart muscle. This can mean that certain areas of the heart do not receive adequate blood flow, and are therefore left damaged. You learned earlier how important the left ventricle is for circulation blood throughout the body. If the left ventricle is damaged by a heart attack, a number of things could happen in addition to the symptoms and complications of a heart attack, which we won't cover in this text.

When heart muscle is damaged from any cause, it's possible that the electrical system of the heart may be damaged also. For example, if the sinus node is damaged, it can cause sinus node dysfunction and possibly lead to abnormally slow or fast heart rhythms. If the AV node is damaged, it could cause heart block, which might result in symptomatic slow heart rates, requiring a pacemaker.

If significant portions of the heart muscle are damaged, the left ventricle may not squeeze as effectively. Remember, the squeeze of the left ventricle is called the LVEF. Damage to the left ventricular muscle may result in a decrease in the LVEF. If the LVEF decreases significantly, the heart may not be able to keep up with the needs of the body, and a condition called **heart failure** may occur. When this occurs, the left ventricle usually gets larger as well (Figure 3). As the left ventricle gets bigger and the squeeze progressively decreases, pressure inside the left ventricle may increase, causing a number of possible symptoms, including shortness of breath with exertion, shortness of breath when lying down, waking up during the night with shortness of breath, swelling of your feet or legs, and sometimes accumulation of fluid in other parts of the body **(edema).**

Congestive heart failure, also referred to by its abbreviation, CHF, is usually first treated with a variety of medications. However, if the medications aren't successful in controlling your symptoms, sometimes a **cardiac resynchronization therapy device** is needed (see Chapter 2). Even if CHF symptoms are well controlled—or perhaps there never were any significant symptoms but the ejection fraction was significantly decreased—your caregiver may recommend that you receive a device called an **implantable cardioverter defibrillator** (ICD). Patients who have an ejection fraction much lower than normal may be at higher risk for having a dangerously fast heart rhythm called **ventricular tachycardia** or **ventricular fibrillation,** the electrical heart rhythms that can cause sudden cardiac arrest (see Chapter 2).

There are many other issues that can impact the electrical system (conduction system) and the plumbing system (coronary arteries) of your heart that we haven't covered here. If your caregiver is describing something that hasn't been explained in this chapter, ask her or him to explain if it is an electrical problem, or a plumbing problem, or both. Don't be afraid to ask questions. Whether the patient is you or a loved one, it's important that you understand what the problem is and what caused it. Ask for educational materials about the medical condition. There is a good chance that your caregiver will either have information available or be able to refer you to a ready and reliable source of information. (Sources of information are also listed later in this book.)

Chapter 2

Types of Devices

PACEMAKERS

A **pacemaker** is a device designed to prevent slow heart rates. It doesn't do anything to prevent fast heart rates, including the most common rhythm abnormality, **atrial fibrillation,** which comes from the top chambers of the heart.

The oldest of all implantable cardiac devices, pacemakers have been available for more than 50 years. Over the years, there have been many variations of the pacemaker, but the basic system includes the pacemaker "can," also known as the **pulse generator,** and the lead or leads that serve as the link between the pacemaker and the heart (Figure 1). The **leads** are often referred to as "wires," but throughout this chapter, we will use the term "leads."

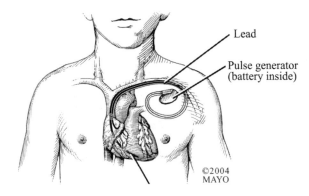

Figure 1. Cartoon of patient with a pacemaker and two leads inside the heart.

The outside of the pulse generator is traditionally made of titanium (Figure 2). Titanium is a metal that almost never results in an allergic reaction or rejection by human tissues. Titanium is also very strong, so there is no need to worry about damaging your device while engaging in almost any routine activity. The pulse generator includes a battery and the **pacemaker circuitry.** The battery is not like common household batteries but is a special battery made of lithium-iodine. This particular type of battery will last for much longer than your household batteries. Another advantage is that when it starts to deplete or wear out, it does so in a very slow and predictable fashion. This is very helpful, as no one wants your pacemaker battery to run out suddenly or unexpectedly. The length of time the batteries will last depends on many things, including how frequently pacing is required and also the electrical characteristics of the lead. However, on average, the pacemaker battery should last 6 to 8 years. Keep in mind that every situation

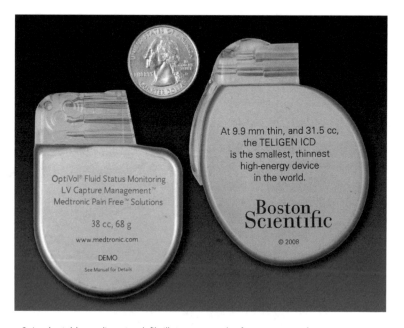

Figure 2. Implantable cardioverter defibrillators; examples from two manufacturers.

is different, and for some patients the pacemaker may last as little as 3 to 4 years or as long as 12 years or more. After your device has been implanted, your physician will be able to give you a more precise estimate based on your particular device, leads, and heart. (See Chapter 6 for more on what to expect after your implant.) When the battery does wear out, the entire device is replaced, not just the battery, because the battery is sealed inside the device, whether it's a pacemaker or a defibrillator.

The pacemaker circuitry is the "brains" of the device and controls all functions of the pacemaker. It is essentially the computer in your device. The circuitry also allows the pulse generator to communicate with an external piece of equipment called the **programmer** (see Chapter 6). With the programmer, the settings or functions of the pacemaker can be altered as needed. This is done completely painlessly in your doctor's office.

The leads consist of one or two **electrodes,** or wires wrapped in insulation (Figure 3). There are many varieties of pacing leads. The end of the lead may have a small screw to attach to the heart wall, called **active fixation** or **screw-in,** or it may have small, flexible tines that get caught in the rough wall of the heart, called **passive fixation.** The lead is usually insulated with

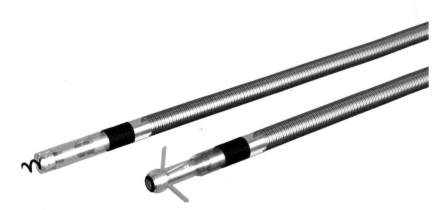

Figure 3. Pacing leads. Used with permission of Medtronic, Inc.

one of two materials, either **polyurethane** or **silicone rubber.** The type of insulation material is not something a patient would need to be aware of or concerned about. If you are the curious type and want to know what type of insulation your leads have, either ask your clinician or simply call your device company. They are usually very helpful and often enjoy talking to patients directly. (See Appendix 1 for device company contact information.)

There are two other terms that patients may hear caregivers use related to the leads. A **unipolar** lead is a single wire with insulation around it, and a **bipolar** lead is one that has two wires that are insulated from each other and from the outside.

The pacemaker may be connected to one or two leads. A pacemaker that uses one lead is called a **single-chamber pacemaker,** and a pacemaker that uses two leads is called a **dual-chamber pacemaker.** A single-chamber device is most commonly one in which the lead is placed in the lower chamber of the heart, specifically on the right side of the heart (i.e., right-ventricular lead placement). This would be called a **VVI** or **VVIR pacemaker.** It is also possible to have a single-chamber system with the lead placed in the right atrium, **AAI** or **AAIR** designation, but these are not commonly used. A dual-chamber device uses leads in both the top and bottom chambers of the heart, usually the right atrium and right ventricle. This would most commonly be called a **DDD** or **DDDR system.** (See Appendix 2 for a more detailed description of pacemaker codes such as these.)

IMPLANTABLE CARDIOVERTER DEFIBRILLATORS (ICDs)

An implantable cardioverter defibrillator (ICD) is a device that's designed to treat life-threatening rapid heart rates, also called **tachycardias** or **tachyarrhythmias.** (ICDs are sometimes simply referred to as "defibrillators" or even "defibs" for short.) All ICDs include a pacemaker, and are thus slightly larger in size than a pacemaker device by itself (Figure 4). The reason a

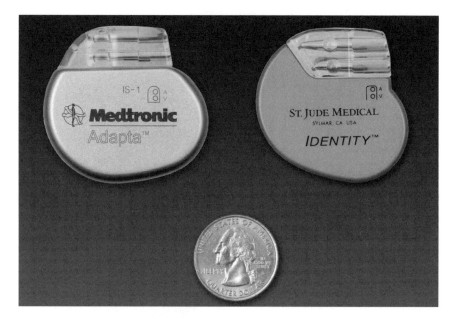

Figure 4. Two different pacemakers, photographed with an American quarter to give an appreciation for their small size.

pacemaker is included is that even if the patient has no history of a problematic slow heart rate, it's possible that the heart rate could be slow for a few seconds immediately after a shock is delivered. The pacemaker is there for those occasions when it may be temporarily needed.

ICDs have been available for about 25 years and are frequently used today. The system consists of the ICD "can" or pulse generator and, like pacemakers, may be a **single-** or **dual-chamber system.**

ICDs are capable of treating tachycardias in two basic ways. If the patient has a very rapid but regular rhythm coming from the lower chambers of the heart, **ventricular tachycardia** (Figure 5), the rhythm might be stopped by rapidly pacing the heart, for example at rates of 250 or 300 beats per minute, for very short bursts. This is called **ATP,** or **antitachycardia pacing.** The ATP bursts are painless, and usually the patient is not even aware that they're occurring.

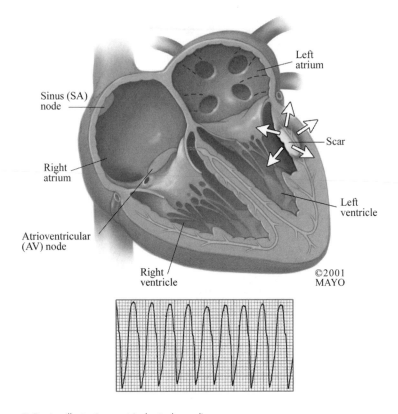

Figure 5. Tracing illustrating ventricular tachycardia.

If the heart rhythm coming from the ventricles is completely erratic and disorganized, it's called **VF**, or **ventricular fibrillation** (Figure 6). With VF, there is no effective "squeeze" or output from the main pumping chambers, and the patient usually loses consciousness and collapses. If not treated quickly, the completely chaotic, unorganized heart rhythm will lead to death. VF may respond to ATP, but it may also require a shock to convert it back to a regular rhythm. Depending on the patient's level of consciousness at the time the shock is delivered, they may or may not be aware of the shock.

The lead used in the ventricle for an ICD system is different from a pacemaker lead. It not only detects abnormal heart rates, but it is also is capable

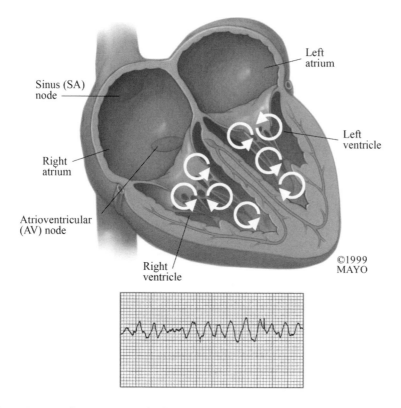

Figure 6. Tracing illustrating ventricular fibrillation.

of delivering a shock directly to the heart. This shock is designed to get the patient out of VT or VF very quickly. In order to accomplish this, the lead has an extra wire (or two) with a section that is not insulated. This allows the electricity from the shock to reach a large portion of the heart directly. These extra wires that are visible on the outside of the lead are called **shocking coils** (Figure 7).

CARDIAC RESYNCHRONIZATION THERAPY (CRT)

Cardiac resynchronization therapy devices (CRT for short) were first approved for use around 2001. (CRT devices are also referred to as **biventricular** or

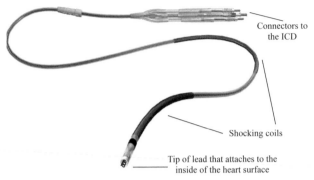

Connectors to
the ICD

Shocking coils

Tip of lead that attaches to the
inside of the heart surface

Figure 7. Defibrillation lead. Used with permission of Medtronic, Inc.

BiV devices.) These devices are used for patients who have a failing heart pump and have symptoms as a result. This "pump failure" is called **congestive heart failure.** There are multiple conditions or criteria that need to be met before a CRT is considered.

In a patient with heart failure, the main pumping chamber (the left ventricle) is often quite large and doesn't squeeze in a uniform way. That is, instead of all walls of the left ventricle contracting at the same time, often, one side of the left ventricle starts to beat before the other side, making the pumping even less effective. With a CRT device, two leads are placed to pace both ventricles—which is where the term BiV (biventricular) originates—instead of just one ventricle, as is the case in a pacemaker or ICD. One ventricular lead is placed in the right ventricle, and another lead is placed in such a way that the outer wall of the left ventricle is also stimulated (Figure 8). By pacing both ventricles as close to 100% of the time as possible, the (ideal) result is that both walls of the left ventricle are stimulated and contract at the same time, improving the efficiency or output of the left ventricle.

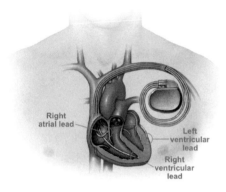

Figure 8. Placement of leads in a CRT device.

Like a pacemaker or ICD, a CRT may be single- or dual-chamber. The device may only have the ability to pace, in which case it's called a **CRT-P** (P = pace), or it may have an ICD incorporated in the system, allowing it to treat fast, potentially dangerous heart rhythms. This is called a **CRT-D** with the "D" referring to "defibrillation" or "ICD"). In the United States and Europe, most CRT systems used are CRT-D devices because patients whose left ventricle is functioning so poorly that they are experiencing heart failure symptoms very often need an ICD also.

Chapter 3

Before Your Device Procedure

The length of time it takes to diagnose your heart condition, the number of doctors you may need to see, and the number and type of tests you may undergo prior to getting your device will depend on the type of problem you are experiencing. Some patients may find themselves feeling totally "normal" one day, and getting a device the next. Other patients may spend months and months trying to find an explanation for their symptoms before they get a device. Because every patient and every diagnosis is unique, the paths to device implant can vary tremendously.

Earlier in this book, we explained the three basic types of cardiac devices that are used: pacemakers, ICDs, and CRT devices. The first step in getting any one of these devices is simply finding the right doctor. The type of doctor who may recommend a device and/or refer you to another doctor for the device procedure will vary. Therefore, it is probably easiest to describe the doctors according to device type.

CHOOSING A DOCTOR

If you are initially seen by your primary care provider, he or she will probably refer you to a **cardiologist.** You may need to see either a general cardiologist or a specialized cardiologist. A cardiologist who has gone on for further training to specialize in heart rhythm problems is called an **electrophysiologist.** If your main problem is one of heart failure, then you may be referred to a cardiologist who has specific training in heart failure. He or she is simply referred to as a **heart failure specialist.**

Finding the appropriate doctor can be accomplished with the help of your usual caregiver, by talking to friends who may have previously had a device implanted, or by looking at reliable sites on the Internet that may provide direction. (For example, the main professional society of electrophysiologists, the Heart Rhythm Society, has information for patients at www.hrsonline .org, as does the professional society for heart failure specialists, the Heart Failure Society of America, at www.hfsa.org.)

TESTING PRIOR TO RECEIVING A DEVICE

Once you have been referred to a physician in the field of cardiology, the path toward diagnosis and implant will continue to vary by device type.

Testing Before Pacemaker Implantation

As described in Chapter 2, a pacemaker is used when the heart rate is too slow and either results in symptoms of **syncope** *(sin-co-pee),* which is the medical term for passing out, or **pre-syncope,** which simply means coming close to passing out. A pacemaker may also be needed if you have specific abnormalities on your heart tracing, the medical term for which is **electrocardiogram,** or ECG (some people also abbreviate this as EKG). These abnormalities indicate that you are at risk for developing a dangerously slow heart rhythm that could cause severe symptoms.

If you've never had an **ECG,** you will definitely have one or more performed (Figure 1). It's a simple test that consists of placing a few electrodes on your chest to record the electrical signals of your heart.

It's also likely that you may have some type of heart rhythm monitoring for a longer period of time. A **Holter monitor,** or ambulatory monitor, is a very small monitor, about the size of a credit card but thicker, that you wear for 24 to 48 hours. A few (two or three) electrodes will be stuck to your chest and connected to the monitor. The monitor can be worn around your neck, hidden under your shirt. The Holter monitor records an ECG the entire time you are wearing it. Your doctor will ask you to keep a diary during the time you are wearing the monitor. You will be asked to record your activities and any symptoms you experience. This allows the doctor to correlate your activities and your symptoms with your heart rate and type of rhythm. If you have symptoms that occur at the same time that your heart rate is

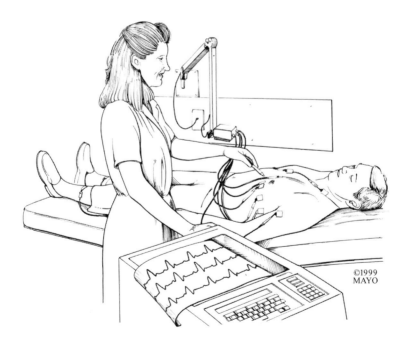

©1999
MAYO

Figure 1. Patient having an electrocardiogram, also called ECG or EKG, performed.

inappropriately slow for a given level of activity, this information may help the caregiver determine whether a pacemaker should be recommended.

If the symptoms you are having are very infrequent—that is, it is unlikely they will occur in the 24 to 48 hours that you would wear the Holter monitor—you may receive an **event recorder** (Figure 2). An event recorder is very similar to a Holter monitor in terms of size and how it is worn. Sometimes event recorders are placed directly on the skin, and other times small electrodes, or "stickies," are placed on the chest wall and connected by small wires to the event recorder.

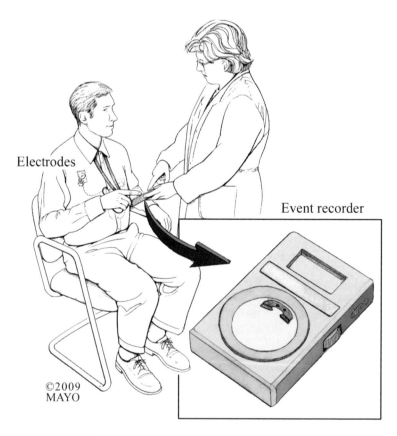

Electrodes

Event recorder

©2009
MAYO

Figure 2. Event recorder.

Like a Holter monitor, the event recorder also records your ECG for the doctors to analyze. The difference is that you keep the event recorder for up to 4 weeks. You put it on yourself every morning. (Generally, you are not asked to wear the monitor during the night unless that is the typical time for your symptoms.) The event recorder is always recording your heart rhythm. However, it only saves a recording of your heart rhythm if you press a button on the activator indicating that you are experiencing symptoms at that time. The recorder will be set up so that when you press the button, it stores a certain number of minutes prior to you pushing the button and a certain number of minutes after pushing the button. Most commonly, you will have been instructed how to call the caregiver's office, or the service that provided the event recorder, to transmit the ECG to them. It is actually possible to transmit this recording over the phone so that your caregiver can review it promptly. If a diagnosis is made on the basis of the recordings that you send in, you will most likely be asked to return to the office to discuss the need for a pacemaker.

Sometimes symptoms can occur because as your heart rate suddenly slows, your blood pressure drops as well. This can be due to something called **vasovagal** (*vās-o-vāg-el*) **syncope** or **neurocardiogenic** (*nur-o-card-e-o-genic*) syncope. This problem occurs when there is an imbalance of the nerves that help control the heart rate and blood pressure. If it is documented that you are having a severe slowing or long pauses of your heart rate, a pacemaker may be indicated, although medications may sometimes be tried first.

To determine whether this problem exists, a **tilt-table study** or **head-up tilt study** may be done (Figure 3). This is not a difficult test for most people. It is done on an outpatient basis, which means you are not admitted to the hospital for the procedure, although it may be performed in a laboratory located in the hospital. You will be asked to go without food the night before the test. When you arrive, you will be connected to an ECG to monitor

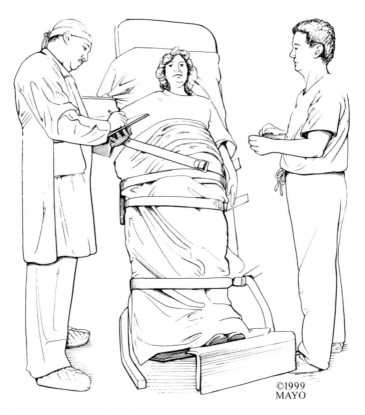

©1999
MAYO

Figure 3. Patient undergoing a tilt-table test.

your heart. You will also wear a blood pressure cuff, and you will receive an IV to give you medications during the test. You will lie flat on a table while your heart rate is monitored and several blood pressure readings are obtained. The special table that you are on will then be tilted up so you are close to a standing position. You will be secured on the table, so there is no concern about slipping off or falling off. You will stay in this tilted position while the nurses or technicians monitor your heart rate and blood pressure. In some individuals with vasovagal or neurocardiogenic syncope, simply being placed in this tilted position during the test will result in symptoms. If that occurs, a definitive diagnosis might be made.

Testing Before an Implantable Cardioverter Defibrillator (ICD) Implant

Before an ICD implant, you may have had ECGs and possibly a Holter monitor or event recorder as well. If any of these document a fast ventricular rhythm, like those previously discussed in Chapter 2 (ventricular tachycardia or ventricular fibrillation), it's possible that no further testing is needed. At other times, if the doctor is suspicious that you had one of these rhythms that resulted in severe symptoms, you may undergo special testing called **electrophysiology testing.** This is an invasive test performed in the hospital. During the test, an electrophysiologist places small **catheters** or tubes in the heart to check out the electrical system of your heart. During this testing, your electrophysiologist will try to actually cause or induce the fast heart rhythm, in order to prove that it really exists. If the rhythm is proven to exist, you will need an ICD.

Sometimes an ICD is recommended when you are determined to be at risk for symptoms, even if you haven't had any yet. Some patients don't survive their first episode of VT or VF, so if at-risk patients can be identified and given an ICD before this first event takes place, it will obviously save many lives. Identifying and implanting patients who are at risk before any symptoms occur is called "primary prevention." (If you have already had an episode where you have collapsed from a fast ventricular rhythm and recovered, placing an ICD is called "secondary prevention.")

The main test used to decide whether you need an ICD, even if you have not experienced any prior symptoms, is an **echocardiogram,** or ultrasound of the heart. This test uses sound waves to make an image of the heart. It looks and feels just like the ultrasound that a pregnant woman would have: a gel is spread on the skin to reduce friction, and an ultrasonic transducer (a handheld device that emits sound pulses) is moved over the heart. The sound pulses bounce painlessly off the heart and return to the receiver, which uses this "echo" to create the image.

An echocardiogram measures how well the main pumping chamber of your heart, the left ventricle, can squeeze out the blood each time it beats. More specifically, the echocardiogram measures the percentage of blood the left ventricle ejects with each beat, which is called the left ventricular ejection fraction (LVEF). A normal LVEF (or EF as it is often called) is about 50 to 60%. From a number of large studies that were done many years ago, we know that patients who have an EF less than 35% are at a greater risk for developing a fast and potentially dangerous ventricular rhythm, and thus very likely to need an ICD.

Many years ago, a push was made to educate everyone to know his or her blood pressure and cholesterol levels. These levels help to show how likely it is that you'll have problems in your heart's plumbing system. Your EF is quite possibly the best measurement to show your risk of having electrical problems in your heart. Therefore, many well-educated patients are starting to track their EF as well.

Testing Before Cardiac Resynchronization Therapy (CRT)

In addition to any combination of the tests already described, you might have been referred to a cardiologist who has special expertise in **congestive heart failure.** If the option of seeing a heart failure specialist hasn't been offered, it's worthwhile to ask your caregiver if that might be a reasonable thing to do in order to get a second opinion. (Your doctor should not be offended by you requesting a second opinion.)

Prior to implantation of the CRT device, some additional blood tests will likely be obtained. You may also have a very simple evaluation called a **"6-minute walk."** True to its name, the 6-minute walk test requires you to see how far you can walk in 6 minutes, noting any symptoms you have during the walk.

QUESTIONS TO ASK THE DOCTOR RECOMMENDING THE PROCEDURE

Many of your questions may be answered throughout the course of the evaluation and testing. However, before entering surgery, you or your family should obtain answers to the following questions:

Prior to pacemaker:

1. What is my diagnosis?
2. Is there any treatment option other than having the pacemaker placed?
3. What will happen if I elect *not* to have a device?

For those of you having specific symptoms:

4. Will the device get rid of my symptoms?
5. With my specific diagnosis, will my insurance company or Medicare recognize this as being needed and cover the cost of the procedure and pacemaker system?
6. What are the possible complications of the procedure? (See Chapter 7.)
7. Is there anything I will no longer be able to do once I get my device? (See Chapter 5.)
8. What follow-up will I have once I get my device, and how long will this device and leads last? (See Chapter 6.)
9. Will I still have to take my medications after I get the device?
10. How will the doctor or the hospital decide which specific device to use?

Prior to ICD:

In addition to the pacemaker questions listed above, you should also ask the following:

1. What is my left ventricular ejection fraction?

2. What are the odds that the ICD will ever be needed?

3. What does a shock feel like? (See Chapters 8 and 9.)

4. Can the ICD be turned off if I develop other medical problems or decide I don't want it on? (See Chapter 10.)

Prior to CRT:

In addition to the pacemaker and ICD questions, you should also ask the following:

1. How likely is it that the CRT device will improve my heart failure symptoms?

2. Does the device just improve symptoms, or does it actually make my heart work more like it's supposed to?

3. Will a CRT have an effect on what medications I am taking or will need to take?

HOW A DEVICE SHOULD BE CHOSEN

As described above, the type of device—pacemaker, ICD, or CRT—will be decided based on your symptoms, your cardiac condition, and the testing performed. Once a decision is made that you need one of these devices, your doctor will choose a specific device from one of the companies that manufactures that specific type of device. There are currently five main companies worldwide that make all three types of devices, although some devices may not be available in all countries.

In general, the doctor who will implant the device will decide which company makes the device most appropriate for you. However, if you have a preference for a specific brand or company based on information from friends and family, you should by all means express that preference to the doctor.

CARDIAC ABLATION BEFORE DEVICE IMPLANTATION

Cardiac ablation refers to a procedure that is very similar to an electro-physiology study during which a very small portion of tissue within the heart is actually destroyed in an effort to control or cure an abnormal heart rhythm. If you undergo an ablation, you won't necessarily need an implantable device too. For example, in some patients who meet the criteria for an ICD device because they have ventricular tachycardia, it may be possible to do an ablation and get rid of the arrhythmia altogether. This would eliminate the need for an ICD.

On the other hand, sometimes an ablation may lead to the need for a device. For example, some patients have atrial fibrillation that leads to an unacceptably fast pulse or ventricular rate. If the heart rate can't be controlled by one of several therapies, the caregivers may suggest that these patients have a procedure called an **AV node ablation.** In this procedure, the electrical connection between the top and bottom chambers of the heart is destroyed so that the unacceptably fast heart rates can no longer occur. However, doing this makes the heart beat too slowly, so these patients will require a pacemaker, and will likely always be dependent on the pacemaker to keep their heart beating at a normal rate. In these cases, the doctor is offering the patient options: exchanging a life-threatening condition (atrial fibrillation) that can't be controlled by other means for a less dangerous condition (bradycardia) that can be controlled with a device.

Whether cardiac ablation is a procedure that should be considered is another question you can ask your caregiver in your appointments prior to surgery.

PREPARING FOR THE DEVICE PROCEDURE

Once your questions are answered and you are scheduled for the procedure, you should receive a few pre-surgical instructions. First, you will need to go without food or liquids after midnight the night before the procedure. To be clear, this means *no food and no water at all*. This is done to prevent any potential complications from having food or fluids in the stomach. The main concern is that if you were to get nauseated and vomit, stomach contents could get into the lungs, which can be a real problem. There may be an exception made for taking certain medications. Ask the caregiver who talks to you about surgery whether you should take your morning medications the day of the procedure. Some will suggest that you take your pills with as small an amount of water as possible, but others may prefer that you wait until after the procedure to take your medications. Do not assume that taking the medications is OK; ask first.

Medications and Surgery

A few specific medications require discussion:

- **Coumadin (warfarin).** If you are on this blood thinner, be sure to ask ahead of time whether you should discontinue the medication. Some implant centers require that you stop it far enough in advance that your blood returns to a normal ability to clot. Depending on the reason you are on warfarin, your caregivers may place you on an injectable blood thinner until the day before the procedure. If this is the method used, you will require the injectable blood thinner after surgery as well, until you have taken warfarin long enough for your blood to become thin again (meaning, long enough for your INR test results to rise). Other implant centers will allow the implant to be done as long as the INR is not too high (that is, the blood is not too thin, which could cause excessive bleeding during surgery and slow down healing afterward).

- **Pradaxa (dabigatran).** This newer medication may be used instead of warfarin in some patients. It also thins the blood, but does not require blood tests to determine the dose. Most patients require the same dose of the medication and currently are required to take it twice a day. If you are on this medication, you will need to talk to your doctor before the procedure to find out if and when they want you to alter the medication dose.

- **Aspirin.** Some patients take a daily dose of aspirin instead of anti-clotting drugs. Most implant centers will have you continue your aspirin, but be sure to ask ahead of time whether you should stop taking it for a period before surgery and especially on the day of surgery.

- **Plavix (clopidogrel)** or similar drugs. Plavix and related drugs affect the cells (platelets) that help your blood to clot. Again, ask your doctor whether you should continue taking this medication prior to surgery. The answer may depend on when it was started and why you are taking it.

- **Diuretics or "water pills" such Lasix (furosemide) and Dyazide (hydrochlorothiazide).** If you normally take a water pill in the morning, you might consider waiting to take it after your procedure, but you will need to talk to your doctor to find out if this is okay. Unlike blood thinners, diuretics don't pose a safety concern. Your doctor might suggest halting your diuretic only for your convenience, so that you don't have to go to the bathroom frequently during the procedure.

- **Insulin.** If you have diabetes and are using insulin to control your blood sugar, ask your doctor whether it should be taken the morning of the procedure. It may also be useful to ask your endocrinologist or diabetes educator to consult with your caregivers. Because you will be fasting and your blood sugar may be lower than usual, many centers would suggest you not take it the morning of the procedure or take a reduced dose.

- **Glucophage (metformin).** Contrast material or dye is sometimes needed during a device implant. Because there can be an interaction between metformin and contrast material, ask your doctor whether you should discontinue the Glucophage. Some caregivers will prefer that this drug be stopped 1 to 2 days prior to your procedure.

The Day of Surgery

Most centers will give you a **surgery time** and an **arrival time.** It is important to arrive at your arrival time, even if it seems excessively early. There is often quite a bit of preparation to be done, which does take some time. The caregiver who talks with you prior to the device implant may give you a special type of anti-bacterial soap to bathe with prior to the procedure as well. If not, simply plan your morning so that you have time to take a shower, using your regular soap, before you leave for the hospital.

A family member or friend should plan on coming with you to the hospital and be available to drive you home when you're released. Do not assume that you will be released on the same day. Some hospitals will send you home the afternoon or evening of the procedure, and others will have you stay overnight. Both are accepted practices, and may vary depending on any other health issues you do or do not have as well. So when planning for transportation, be sure you either ask ahead of time when you'll be released, or make plans for each contingency.

Some centers will include an educational session while you are in the hospital as well. This may happen before your procedure, but often occurs after. Either way, it is wise for a family member to be present for this teaching session for a few reasons. First, patients are often groggy after receiving anesthesia and may be unable to remember instructions. Second, it's always a good idea for more than one person to receive education about the device. If two people hear it, it's more likely that at least one of you will remember the details.

Before the Procedure

Once you sign in and fill out the usual insurance forms and other paper-work, you will be taken to a preoperative preparation area. Here, several people, including the person who will administer your anesthesia, will ask you many questions to prepare for the surgery. You will also get an IV inserted and will be hooked up to an ECG and a blood pressure cuff to monitor your vital signs.

Depending on your medications, you may also need to have blood drawn to ensure that it is safe to proceed with the surgery. Waiting for the results can also take some time. In fact, it's not unusual to spend a few hours in the preoperative preparation area, so you may want to bring a book or a friend to keep your mind busy and away from unnecessary worry.

Before starting the procedure, the local area around the incision site will be shaved and scrubbed with some special soap. This is sometimes done in the procedure room itself after you are asleep, or in the preoperative area, or both. Finally, and quite possibly the most important thing you can do for your own comfort, is make sure to use the restroom just before they come to take you to the procedure room, which can be either an operating suite or an electrophysiology lab.

During the Procedure

Once inside, you will be again be hooked up to a blood pressure cuff and an ECG before any anesthesia can be given. If you are nervous about pos-sible pain, simply ask that you begin some type of anesthesia before any part of the procedure begins. This is almost always done, but it sometimes helps patients feel better to remind their caregiver that they are particularly nervous. Don't be afraid to admit your fears as well. Fear is an emotion experienced by many people before surgery. Often your caregiver can give you some medications once in the procedure room to relax you.

Restrictions After the Implant

Before surgery, you should be informed about any restrictions that will follow the implant so that you can make necessary preparations. Restrictions are usually minimal, but it is important that you carefully follow any instructions your healthcare team gives you. Normal restrictions after device implant include the following:

Driving. You will be instructed not to drive for some period of time after the procedure if you are having new leads placed. (If you are just having your device changed because the previous device has reached a stage where the battery is depleted, you may not have new leads placed. In this case, as long as your leads are not manipulated or replaced, your driving will probably not be restricted for any substantial length of time.)

Driving restriction is primarily a medical-legal or liability issue. If you were involved in an accident shortly after the procedure, someone might suggest that a malfunction of the device led to you having the accident. Even though your device management team could usually prove that the device was functioning normally, it's best to avoid driving right after implant. Different hospitals recommend different lengths of restrictions. After a pacemaker, driving is usually restricted for 10 to 14 days. After a defibrillator, if you have never had any symptoms like passing out, then the restriction may be only 10 to 14 days. If you have passed out as a result of a fast heart rhythm, driving may be prohibited for 3 to 6 months or longer, depending on whether you continue to have symptoms. (For more on driving with an ICD, see Chapter 5.)

Arm motion on the implant side. Most centers doing implants will suggest that you limit the motion of the arm on the side of the procedure for at least 4 weeks. This is to help protect the newly placed leads from moving. It is common for you to be told to restrict the motion of the arm on the same side as the device implant to no higher than shoulder level. Some places will send you home with a sling to be worn loosely as a reminder to limit your arm motion. It is important that you continue moving your arm as allowed, however. Completely immobilizing your arm could lead to shoulder problems.

Hunting or shooting. If you are a hunter or marksman, you should avoid shooting the gun from the side of the device because you don't want the gun to recoil on the device itself. (Firing pistols may still be possible as long as you are able to conform to the restrictions on arm motions while healing.) If the ability to shoot a rifle or shotgun is important to your quality of life, discuss it with the doctor prior to the procedure. This may alter where the doctor places the device. There are almost always options available to allow you to continue to enjoy your sport.

Use of power tools or heavy equipment. There aren't many things in the environment that will interfere with your device. However, it's possible that certain power tools could cause interference. For example, chainsaws, welding equipment, and close contact with a large engine could possibly interfere with your device function. If you have specific hobbies or work-related activities that involve power equipment or heavy machinery, you need to discuss this with your doctor prior to the procedure. But again, if you discuss it with your doctor, some precautions can usually be taken to allow you to continue in many of these hobbies.

Household appliances. There is no issue with normally functioning appliances. The days of microwave ovens causing pacemaker problems are gone. However, faulty or malfunctioning household appliances could have an effect on your device. If you know something isn't working normally, and especially if you or a family member has ever received a shock from the appliance, avoid using it.

If you are concerned about any specific activity that might be affected by having the device, it's better to ask about it before the procedure. In addition to asking the doctor, you can call the patient service line of the major companies. (See Appendix 1.) Other than the restrictions mentioned above, it's unlikely there are things you would have to give up, but it's always better to ask and know ahead of time if there are any concerns. If there are activities that you will have to give up after your device implant, be sure to understand what your options are. You need to understand what will happen if you elect not to get the device. In some instances, you might still not be allowed to do the activity you desire because of your heart problem. (For more on restrictions after the device, see Chapter 5.)

TAKE TIME TO FEEL COMFORTABLE ABOUT GETTING THE DEVICE

There are some situations when a pacemaker or defibrillator is needed urgently. However, for most of you, there will be time to get your questions answered and think it through. In the less common situation where you need the support of a pacemaker urgently, your doctors will place what is called a temporary pacemaker. This type of pacemaker is outside your body and connected to a wire that is temporarily placed in a vein and positioned in your heart.

If you find yourself in a situation where you haven't had time to think things through and feel comfortable with the device, be proactive and ask the doctor if it is really such an emergency that you can't take time to get your questions answered.

Chapter 4

Inside the Procedure Room (Operating Room)

If you've never had surgery before, you may not know what to expect. This chapter describes what you may expect to experience when you go in for your device implant.

PREOPERATIVE PREPARATIONS

As described in the previous chapter, by the time you are taken into the room where your device will be implanted, you will likely already have an intravenous (IV) line in place.

When you are taken into the procedure room, it may seem very cool. The room temperature is often kept cool because the medical personnel doing the implant are wearing a sterile gown over their hospital "scrub" suits as well as an apron made of lead, which is often heavy and hot, as well as a mask, head covering, and eye protection. If you are too cold, tell the nurses or technicians in the room. It's possible to have extra blankets put over you while the team is getting everything else ready.

After you're wheeled into the procedure room, you will be transferred to the procedure table. There will be a lot of equipment in the room, including monitoring equipment and x-ray equipment (Figure 1). The table may be very firm, narrow, and somewhat uncomfortable. There may also be straps attached to the table that are placed around you. They shouldn't be tight. The straps are there for your safety, given the narrow design of the table. It is usually preferable that you lie with your head fairly flat on the table. If you are uncomfortable this way, ask whether you might be able to get a small pillow or a folded blanket placed under your head.

Before anything else is done, even if you've been asked many times already, you may again be asked to state your name and your birth date. This is only a precaution to make sure the right patient is getting the right procedure. You may also hear the team in the procedure room take a "pause," during which they again state your name, the procedure to be done, and

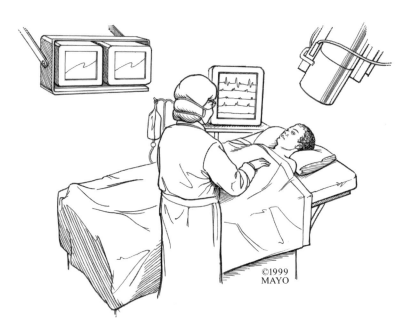

Figure 1. Patient in the operating room, before the chest is scrubbed and the monitoring wires are put in place.

the location where the device will be placed. These are all safeguards to prevent mistakes.

Sticky pads will be placed on your chest so your heart rate and rhythm can be monitored. Frequently, larger sticky pads are placed on the front and back of your chest. These pads can be used to correct an abnormal heart rhythm or possibly to pace the heart if an abnormally slow or fast heart rate should occur during the procedure.

Oxygen will be provided to you throughout the procedure. Sometimes an oxygen mask is put over your mouth and nose, but it's more common that a small tube is placed in such a way that two small, soft nasal prongs send oxygen directly into your nose. A device will also be connected to your finger or toe, or sometimes your ear, to monitor the amount of oxygen in your blood. Oxygen is used only to ensure that your oxygen levels remain normal while you are sedated. Once you are sedated, your breathing is more shallow, which may cause oxygen levels to drop if no oxygen were provided.

The next part of the preparation involves getting the skin clean and creating a very clean and sterile environment as a precaution to prevent an infection. Prior to these next steps, if you have any urge to urinate, let the nurse or technician know. It's much easier for you to use a bedpan or urinal before all of the sterile drapes are in place.

The area where the device will be implanted, usually your upper chest, will be "prepped" or made clean. Men must usually be shaved on the side where the device will be implanted, and all patients are scrubbed with a special anti-bacterial soap of some type. Once your chest is scrubbed, sterile drapes will be placed around the area where the device will be implanted. This will usually involve the drapes or towels covering your face. This may make some people feel closed-in or claustrophobic. The drapes can usually be pulled up in such a way that they are not directly on your face.

Frequently, there will be a nurse or anesthetist positioned close to your head, whom you will be able to see. That individual will be monitoring your blood pressure and heart rate, and will probably also be giving you medications in your IV. These medications will keep you comfortable and may make you sleep. If anything is bothering you—if the drapes are making you feel claustrophobic or you are having discomfort or feel short of breath—tell the caregiver closest to you, and he or she will work to make you feel more comfortable.

For some procedures, your doctor will want another catheter placed in one of your arteries, most commonly at your wrist, to allow continuous measurement of your blood pressure. Often this catheter is placed after you have already been given some medication to help you relax. Once in place, this catheter is very similar to having another IV line. The main difference is that when it's removed, your caregivers may want to apply pressure to the site for longer than they would for a normal IV.

THE ACTUAL PROCEDURE

Next, the area where the incision will be made is injected with a topical anesthetic or "numbing" medicine, most commonly lidocaine. This is very similar to the novocaine your dentist uses. Between the topical anesthetic and the intravenous medications you are receiving, you shouldn't experience any discomfort. If you do, tell someone! You may experience a pressure or tugging sensation at times. This is normal, but it should not be painful.

Once the area is numb and you are completely comfortable or even sleeping, an incision will be made. Most often, the incision is about an inch below your collarbone (clavicle) and is roughly 2 to 4 inches long. The exact size of the incision will depend on what device is being implanted. A pacemaker requires the smallest incision, and an ICD or CRT device for heart failure will require a little bigger incision.

Inside the Procedure Room (Operating Room)

Under your skin is a layer of fat, and below that is the muscle. The device will usually be placed between the fat and the muscle. Once the doctor has reached that area, he or she will make a space large enough to allow the device to fit. The space between the fat and muscle is usually easy to open up and only takes a few minutes. This process is often referred to as "making the pocket" in which the device will reside. Less commonly, the device will be placed under the muscle. Sometimes this is done in smaller children or adults who are very thin and don't have much fat to cover and protect the device. In some patients, placing the device under the muscle may also be cosmetically preferred. However, it takes more time and requires the expertise of a doctor who has experience in placing the device under the muscle. For the majority of adults, implanting the device above the muscle is optimal and cosmetically acceptable. Recovery is also less painful when the physician doesn't have to cut into the muscle.

After the pocket is made, the leads need to be placed in the heart. There are large veins located just under and slightly below the collar bone. A needle is placed into one of these veins, and then a thin wire is threaded through the needle and directed into the chambers of the heart. The needle is then removed. The doctor can then put another straw-like tube or sheath over the wire and then remove the wire. With the tube or sheath in place, the doctor can pass the lead or leads through the tube and into the heart chambers. The tube can then be pulled away, and all that remains is the lead going into the large veins that lead into the heart.

Guided by x-ray, the doctor will move the lead into the correct place in the heart. Sometimes one lead will be placed, sometimes two—and for CRT devices used to treat heart failure, three leads might be needed. Once the doctor has the leads in a good spot, he or she will secure them in place. The leads inside the heart often have a small screw on the end of them that actually screws into the heart muscle. If you're awake enough that you're hearing any of the conversation, and you hear the doctor ask for a screwdriver, don't be alarmed. He or she is asking for a tiny tool that is used at the end of the lead to make the screw on the other end go into the heart muscle. You will not be able to feel this happening, and it doesn't damage the heart.

When the leads are secured in place, the doctor and the nurse or technician will do measurements on the lead to make sure they have a good electrical connection. Testing this electrical connection is very important for ensuring that the device can function normally. If the measurements aren't good, it might be necessary to move the lead and try again. Most of the time, it doesn't take too long to place leads in the right atrium and right ventricle, although lead placement times can vary quite a bit.

If you are having a CRT device placed for heart failure, another lead will be placed in one of the veins of the heart. The doctor will get to the vein through the heart chambers, but the vein is located on the outside of the left ventricle. This lead can take significantly longer to place. These leads are also different in that they aren't secured with a screw. Instead, they are made secure by being placed at an angle that wedges them into the vein, or using some other mechanism that helps hold them in place.

When all of the leads are in place and the doctor is satisfied with the electrical measurements, the leads are sewn down to the muscle near the location where the device will be placed. Following this, the leads are connected to the device. The doctor will double-check to make sure they are securely locked into the appropriate receptacle on the device.

The pacemaker, ICD, or CRT will then be placed in the "pocket" space that was formed between the chest wall muscle and the fat above it. Excess lead may be coiled behind the device and also placed in the pocket.

Using the external programmer—the equipment used to check the device and make changes in the device settings—the electrical measurements may be repeated. If you're having a pacemaker implanted, the procedure is almost over. The only thing left to do is close the incision.

If you're having a defibrillator placed, there may be one additional step. Since the purpose of a defibrillator is to recognize a dangerously fast heart rhythm and then treat the heart rhythm with a shock, your doctor will often want to test this function before the procedure is completed. This is just a way to double-check that the device is able to appropriately detect and treat an arrhythmia. This procedure is called **defibrillation threshold testing,** often abbreviated as **DFT.** DFT defines the amount of energy or "threshold" that it takes to successfully shock the bad heart rhythm back to a normal heart rhythm.

For the few minutes that this test is conducted, you will be put into a deeper sleep with anesthesia to ensure that you do not feel the shock that will be delivered. Using the programmer, the doctor will use the device to cause your heart to go into ventricular fibrillation while you are closely monitored. Once the fast heart rhythm has been induced, the ICD will treat the rhythm with a shock, and the doctor will note how much energy it took to shock the fast rhythm back to a regular rhythm and how accurately the ICD recognized the abnormal rhythm. This procedure allows both you and the physician to leave the operating room fully satisfied that your device is working properly, ready and able to save you from any life-threatening rhythms that may occur.

If DFT testing is performed, the incision will be closed after testing is complete. There are different ways to close the incision, including stitches, staples, and glue. Sometimes combinations of these closure methods are used. Each doctor or hospital will have their own preferences, and you should ask your caregivers after the procedure how the incision was closed and whether any stitches will need to removed.

Once the incision is closed, you will be taken to a recovery room until the drugs you have been given start to wear off and you are awake. Depending on the hospital's protocol, you may be transferred to a hospital room or an outpatient area. Some hospitals do the device implants as outpatient procedures and send people home on the same day. Patients are then expected to come back to an outpatient area the next day to check the incision and the device function. Other hospitals will keep the patient overnight and conduct the device check in the hospital the next morning.

Overall procedure times will vary widely. A quick, straightforward single-chamber pacemaker could be done in as little as 30 minutes, while a more complicated three-lead CRT system could take many hours. You and your family members also need to know that in addition to the actual procedure time, the length of time you will be away from your room also includes the preparatory time and the recovery time. This could easily add an hour on the front end and an hour after the procedure. Finally, have your family ask where they should wait and how they can get updates on your progress.

Finally, before you leave the hospital, you should receive instructions regarding when you can shower and resume normal activities, and about your first follow-up appointment. Most facilities have educational protocols for pacemaker or ICD implants that will teach you about your device, any restrictions you may have, and the follow-up plan (see Chapter 6).

Chapter 5

What Next?
After Your Procedure

COMING OUT OF SURGERY

After your surgery, you will likely be sore. However, most patients coming out of surgery complain less about pain around their incision and more about general soreness. After lying still and flat on a hard table for what could be several hours, patients often have quite a few aches and pains. Usually, your caregiver will try to get you up and about within a few hours. Even a short walk to the restroom can help alleviate the stiffness that you may be feeling.

The main restriction will be regarding movement of your arm and shoulder on the side of the device implant. In fact, you will probably be given a sling to wear loosely for the first days, or even weeks, following the implant procedure. This sling is mainly there as a reminder to keep your arm and shoulder fairly still. Before you are discharged from the hospital, you may be instructed to wear your sling only at night to help you not to move your arm excessively while sleeping. Other institutions will instruct you to wear your sling during the day as well. Whichever the case, it is important to make sure you don't stop using your shoulder completely, as that can lead to a problem called **frozen shoulder.** As a general rule of thumb, keep your elbow below your nipple line at all times. Any extreme stretching (such as reaching up to a high shelf) should be avoided. You can use your opposite arm and shoulder normally. For this reason, if you are right-handed, your doctor will probably implant the device on your left side, and vice versa.

As explained earlier in the book, the leads that are placed in your heart go through a vein that is just below your collarbone. During surgery, the leads are gently affixed to the heart and remain stable until, over several weeks, scar tissue naturally forms around them. However, excessive arm and shoulder motion on the side of the implant could contribute to the leads moving out of place. If this were to happen, you might need another surgery to reposition the leads. Because of this risk, you will be given a lifting restriction of about 5 pounds. A gallon of milk weighs about 8 pounds and is a good reference to keep in mind. You will also be given instructions on restricting the movement of the arm on the side of the implant. These restrictions usually last for 4 to 8 weeks, depending on the physician, the procedure, and the patient. After your 4 to 8 weeks are up, you can go back to using your arm and shoulder just as you did before you got your device.

If your procedure was simply a generator change (also called a "battery change"), you may not have any of the above restrictions on movement. (Note: Even though it is often called a "battery change," the battery itself is not taken out and replaced. Instead, the pacemaker is detached from the leads and exchanged for a brand new pacemaker.) If no new leads were added to your system, you should not have any arm movement restrictions. If your leads have been in long enough to build up scar tissue, then there is less concern about them falling out of place, and you therefore won't be given a sling.

What Next? After Your Procedure

Before leaving the hospital, you should also receive educational materials. These materials may come from the hospital, the device manufacturer, or both. Your first follow-up appointment will be scheduled for you. This first follow-up appointment is generally called a **wound check.** At this appointment, your caregiver will check your incision for signs of infection.

It is important that you also do your part in preventing and watching for any infection. Follow all the instructions given to you in the hospital, and check your incision daily for redness, swelling, and any draining. Let your caregiver know if you are concerned about the appearance of the incision or area around the incision. You will also be given instructions on how to care for your wound. These instructions will vary according to the preferences of the hospital where your device was implanted and the preferences of the doctors and nurses involved with your care. Most recommend keeping the incision dry for 1 to 2 days and, when you do bathe, that you allow water to run over the incision but avoid scrubbing it until it is no longer tender. Also, if small adhesive strips called "steri-strips" were placed over the incision, you will probably be instructed not to remove them until they start to come loose on their own. If they are still present after 2 weeks, you should peel them off.

Some hospitals will use oral antibiotics after the procedure. You will probably be sent home with some pain medicine. Most patients generally need prescription pain medicines for less than a week, sometimes only a few days. If you continue to experience any significant pain after this time, notify your caregiver of the excess pain.

If you've had only a generator change, you may need very little pain medication. In a generator change procedure, the physician will often attempt to cut over the previous incision. (If this is important to you, don't be afraid to ask the physician before the procedure is this is possible.) This can have cosmetic benefits by minimizing the chances of you having another scar. In general, patients experience less pain after a generator change than after the first implant because the skin has already stretched out to make room for the device and the body has formed a thick scar or **fibrosis** around the device.

Before you leave the hospital, you will also be given a temporary ID card. This is a credit card–sized piece of paper that contains detailed information about your device and leads. It is a good idea to keep this with you at all times. Most patients simply put it in their purse or wallet. If you ever need to go to the emergency room or you are traveling away from your usual doctor, this card will be helpful to the physicians treating you.

Within about a month of leaving the hospital, you should receive a permanent version of this card in the mail. It will be sent to you directly from your device manufacturer. This card will be plastic and much more durable. Make sure to check the card for any errors. If you notice any, call the phone number on the card to report the error, and the manufacturer will send you a new card.

ELECTROMAGNETIC INTERFERENCE: SOME DO'S AND DON'TS

Although devices have certainly improved over the years, and now require far fewer restrictions than they used to, there are still a few restrictions to be aware of. You will be instructed about specific sources of **electrical and/ or magnetic interference** that could confuse or interfere with the function of your device. Interference with a pacemaker could inhibit the pacemaker so that it doesn't pace when it should. Interference with an ICD could make the device think you are having a fast heart rhythm when you aren't and could lead to an inappropriate shock. Keep in mind that patients who are diligent with their follow-up, either through home monitoring or in-office visits, are less likely to experience device or lead problems that would possibly make them more susceptible to issues with interference.

Electromagnetic fields can be found in almost all electronic devices, including **cell phones, iPods,** and **power tools.** The good news is that the electromagnetic fields created by these devices are rarely strong enough to interfere with your device. You may be instructed to use a cell phone on the ear opposite your device and to avoid placing an activated cell phone in a breast pocket situated over your device. As a general rule of thumb, keep electrical devices at least 6 inches away from your device. This may be a little overcautious, but is certainly a safe practice.

Some other issues deserve mention. **Anti-theft devices** at the doors of many department stores or libraries generally won't cause any trouble. However, avoid stopping and standing inside these machines or leaning against them. Instead, simply walk through at a normal pace. The expression used is *"Don't linger... don't lean."*

Airport metal detectors generally will not cause any interference with your device. However, because the metal in the device could set off the metal detector, it's better to simply tell the security personnel about your pacemaker or ICD. They will give you a "pat down" instead. Don't be embarrassed to notify airline personnel of your device. They deal with patients with implanted medical devices every day.

There are a few things outside the hospital environment that are potentially a more significant source of interference to the device. The most common of these is arc welders. If you use an arc welder as part of your job or hobby, discuss this with your caregivers. They will probably want to know the power or amperage of your welding equipment. Depending on their experience, your type of device, and your particular heart rhythm problem, they will decide whether welding is something you need to avoid. The same issue exists with chainsaw use. Talk with your caregivers about the specifics of the equipment you want to use, and they will advise you about the safest way to proceed.

There is some equipment in the hospital or clinic setting that could interfere with device function. Different types of **ablation equipment** and procedures, cardioversion, surgery or other procedures when **electrocautery** is used, some **radiation treatments**, some **chiropractic equipment**, and a type of imaging called **magnetic resonance imaging (MRI)** may all interfere with your device's functioning. In general, make sure you tell your medical providers that you have a device before any medical procedure is performed. They will take the proper precautions so that you can still undergo most of these procedures safely. (The most common exception would be MRI, which may not be possible to perform. There are new pacemaker systems that should be safe for MRI, but unless you've specifically been told that you have a device *and* leads that are safe for MRI, it may not be possible to undergo this type of imaging.)

Finally, there is a very small number of patients who may have to make significant lifestyle changes after device implant. For example, patients with implanted heart devices are usually prohibited from working as airplane pilots or commercial vehicle drivers. Restrictions may also be placed on individuals who have to climb and work on electrical power lines. Making a lifestyle or occupational change like this may be a big adjustment. However, it is important to keep things in perspective. There are patients who refuse a device because they are concerned about the restrictions they will face after implant. They lose sight of the fact that overall, they would be safer receiving the device. Remember that it is the underlying heart condition that usually causes major life changes, not the device per se. Any type of illness can cause disruptions in your life, and this can be difficult to cope with for anyone. (For more on this, see Chapter 9.)

CAN I DO THAT?

Once your initial 4- to 8-week restriction on lifting and reaching is over, you should be able to resume your usual activities. In fact, there are very few things that having a device will prevent you from doing. However, it is possible that the heart conditions that led to you receiving a device could result in your doctor placing some restrictions on your activities. A device won't keep you from running a marathon or playing ice hockey or even skydiving. However, severe heart disease may keep you from some, or all, of the above activities. It is important to talk to your physician about what you can and cannot do. Some of you may be instructed to exercise frequently. Whatever the case may be, it is important to understand what you can do to help improve your overall health condition; as always, talk to your doctor.

Like the vast majority of ICD, pacemaker, and CRT patients, once the incision has fully healed, you will probably forget it is even there. It's likely that no one would know you even have a device unless you choose to tell them about it. Generally, just getting a device doesn't have to slow you down.

TWO QUESTIONS

There are two questions about daily activities that device patients ask most frequently. They are: "Can I continue to be intimate with my spouse or significant other?" and "Can I drive?" While we will discuss the intimacy issues further in Chapter 9, the simple answer to the first question is yes—if you could do so before your device implant, you can do so following the device implant. The driving issue isn't quite as straightforward and requires further discussion.

In the short term after your implant, you will not be allowed to drive. Immediately after your implant, the driving restriction is placed because you have received anesthesia and pain medications. The length of time your driving is restricted may vary depending on whether you have a history of passing out, the type of device you receive, and the other details of your medical condition. If you have passed out from an arrhythmia, or your doctor determines that you are at an increased risk for passing out, this restriction may last for months. Discuss this issue with your caregiver if you have any concerns. They will be aware not only of your specific situation, but also of the laws that apply in your state of residence. Most states have regulations regarding driving restrictions if you have a history of passing out. The restriction is typically for 3 to 6 months, perhaps longer if you have recurrent episodes of passing out.

Even if you are given permission to resume driving, you may be hesitant and concerned about driving safely with an ICD. For many people, driving represents independence and is an important part of returning to a normal life after device implant. If this is true for you, it may help to focus on the positive aspects of driving with an ICD instead of the negatives. Remember that since you have been identified as someone who is at risk for a life-threatening arrhythmia, you are much safer driving with an ICD than you would be driving without one. Even if you have never had an arrhythmia or an episode of passing out, there is always a chance of this occurring. Patients who experience arrhythmias and are not fortunate enough to have an ICD will likely lose consciousness. Clearly, this situation becomes more dangerous for the patient and others around them if it occurs while the patient is driving.

Driving with an ICD is a safer situation because the odds of you losing consciousness are decreased. For many patients, the ICD will deliver treatment before consciousness is lost and you will have time to pull over to the side of the road and call for help. It may be comforting to know that research studies have found that ICD patients as a whole are a safer group of drivers than the general public, and that ICD shocks while driving and subsequent fatal car accidents are extremely rare. Hopefully, the fact that you have an ICD will eventually make you and your family members feel safer and more secure about you driving, as opposed to less so.

Of course, every patient is unique and may deal with these issues in different ways. What if you've only had one abnormal heart rhythm 10 years ago? Are you safe to drive? What if you get shocks for dangerous heart rhythms every month, but have never passed out? An open, honest conversation with your caregivers and your family members is usually the only way to make responsible decisions. Among the many things that need to be discussed with your caregiver are your type and rate of abnormal heart rhythms, how your device is programmed, your past heart history, and your current medications. If you find yourself struggling with a decision about driving, make sure that you, your spouse or family, and your physician are all comfortable with you driving before you get behind the wheel again.

PERSONAL STORY

I received my ICD at age 17, after having five episodes of sudden cardiac death, all requiring CPR to save my life. When I got my device, we didn't need to discuss driving much because I knew that every time I had an episode, I felt it coming. I always had about 10 seconds or so from when my heart started racing until I passed out. We (my parents, my doctors, and I) figured this was plenty of time to hit the brakes and pull over should I feel an episode coming on. I had more than 20 arrhythmia episodes over the next 15 years, all of which were similar to the first five episodes. The difference was that now I had my ICD, which would get my heart out of its bad rhythm, either before I passed out or just as I was passing out.

Everything changed one day when I was in my early 30s. I was standing and talking to my brother-in-law when I suddenly felt a little funny. The next thing I knew, I was waking up. Apparently, I had passed out, and about 5 to 10 seconds later, my ICD shocked me. In the days following, we (my wife, my doctors, and I) discussed the issue of driving. However, this time the "driving" discussion was quite different. According to state law, I couldn't drive for 6 months. However, we all wondered if I should continue to drive after that. What if it happened again?

After the 6-month restriction was up, we decided I was okay to drive, with medication and some changes in my device programming. I went back to driving until I passed out a few months later. This time, sitting at home talking on the phone, I lost consciousness without any notice. Once again, legally, I couldn't drive for 6 months, but again, I asked myself—what about after that? It seemed to me that 6 months was just an arbitrary number set by some lawmaker. I was just as likely to have an event 6 months and 1 day later as 6 months later.

This time, my doctor was much less comfortable with me driving, and my wife hated the idea of me driving again. We now had two baby daughters, and she didn't think it was worth the risk. Deep down, I knew they were right, and I felt that I probably shouldn't drive. However, not driving would mean a career change and other major lifestyle adjustments, especially given that we lived in a rural area without any public transportation.

Fortunately, my wife and doctor basically took the decision out of my hands, and I haven't driven in several years. Although it was undoubtedly the most difficult adjustment of my life, it all worked out. I've adjusted. I don't know what the future holds—perhaps I'll get to drive again one day—but I've learned to live without it. Although I've had to give up a few things, all in all I still do the things I love to do. I've adapted. It's amazing how creative you can get when you must.

IS MY DEVICE A CURE?

Sometimes your device may effectively be a cure to your heart problem. This is particularly true with some pacemaker patients. Many CRT patients may find an overall improvement in their symptoms and possibly their heart condition as well. For other patients, their device will simply be a safety net to save their life when all else fails. As we've seen many times before in this book, the answer to this question is most often about your particular heart condition and not about the device you receive.

This same principle applies to the often-asked question, "Will the device allow me to stop my medications?" Again, it all depends on your heart condition. Make sure to include this in your list of questions to ask your doctor before you leave the hospital. Some of you may get to discontinue or decrease some medications before going home, while others will actually leave the hospital with more medications.

NEED ANSWERS?

If you have technical questions regarding your device, consider calling the toll-free number provided by your device company. This "Patient Services" phone number will likely be listed on your patient ID card. The device companies are happy to talk with patients who receive their devices, and receiving this type of technical expertise can be quite reassuring.

Finally, if you would like to travel after your implant, the device companies can be a great resource. They can often provide a list of physicians who follow their devices all over the world. Having the name of a physician in another city who will be familiar with your device can be helpful and comforting, especially if you are traveling internationally.

Chapter 6

Follow-Up Care

HOW OFTEN DO I NEED MY DEVICE CHECKED?

One of the most important things that you can do as a device patient is to be diligent with your device follow-up appointments. Your caregiver will decide how often your device needs to be checked depending on your type of device, your health status, and the caregiver's preferences for follow-up. However, as a general guideline, patients with an ICD will usually have their device checked, or "interrogated," about once every 3 to 4 months. The schedule for pacemaker patients will vary a great deal depending on how the follow-up center manages its patients. Anything from monthly checks to checks every 6 months can be typical. The schedule will also depend on what type of follow-up is used (that is, in-office checks or remote transmissions). The follow-up schedule is often a little more intensive for the first several months after implant, however.

Your follow-up appointments are important for monitoring the status of the device and leads. These follow-up visits may reveal issues with your system before they cause you any identifiable problem. However, as the rate of failure in heart devices is quite low, often it's the other information about your heart that the device gathers that can prove most helpful. Pacemakers,

ICDs, and CRT devices monitor every heartbeat of every day. While doing this, they count every single beat and make a note of the abnormal heartbeats. They plot out your heart rates, showing your caregiver how often your device is working and how often your heart is beating (correctly) on its own. Current devices monitor and record a great deal of information, and your caregiver has access to everything stored in the device.

HOW DO YOU CHECK MY DEVICE?

Although your device is under your skin, your caregiver can get information out of your device, or make changes to its settings, with a **programmer.** The programmer is basically a portable desktop computer with a **communication wand** attached. The wand is a small communication tool that can "talk" to your implanted device. It attaches to the programmer with a small cable. By placing the wand directly on top of your device, it can communicate with your implanted device. The wand works through your skin, and usually even works through a few light layers of clothing. Some of the newer devices and programmers are wireless, meaning they don't even need a wand placed over your device. Instead, information is exchanged between the two devices using radio frequency communications and small antennae (Figure 1).

Whether your device is a newer model or an older one, each device has only one particular programmer that is capable of checking the device and making changes. This will depend on which device manufacturer made the device you have. Any caregiver can tell which programmer is needed for you based on the information on your patient identification card. That's another reason it is so important to carry your identification card with you at all times.

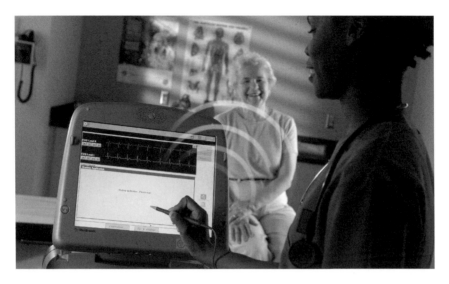

Figure 1. Wireless device interrogation programming can be done at a distance of 6 to 10 feet. Used with permission of Medtronic, Inc.

YOUR DEVICE'S SETTINGS

Within each device there are literally hundreds of features and settings that your caregiver can change. It is beyond the scope of this book to cover them all and describe how they function. Yet it is important to be aware of a few of the basic settings to help you better understand your device. Perhaps the most basic and important settings are the **lower rate limit (LRL)** and the **upper rate limit (URL)**.

Your LRL is the slowest that your device will let your heart beat. This number is usually programmed between 40 and 70, but can vary widely. If set at 70, simply put, your device will not let your heart fall below 70 beats per minute. Therefore, if you know that your device's LRL is set to 70, you should never find your pulse rate much less than that.

The URL is essentially the same thing, but on the fast side. It is the fastest rate that your device is able to pace the heart. The URL of the device doesn't limit the rate your own heart rhythm can go. If you ever take your pulse and find that your heart is beating faster than your URL, this simply means that your heart is choosing to go fast all by itself, without any help from the device. Remember that the pacemaker portion of your device cannot slow down your heart, but can only keep your heart from beating too slowly.

When it comes to slowing down fast rhythms, the only two options available through an implantable device include a special type of pacing therapy or a shock from an ICD. Thus, your caregiver will program your ICD to a fast rate at which some type of therapy will be delivered. This is generally set anywhere between 150 and 200 beats a minute, but again, can vary widely. Once your own heart rate reaches this programmed number, the device will initiate treatment for that fast rhythm. The treatment may be a combination of **rapid pacing therapy** and different-strength shocks. There are many programmable options for how many rounds of therapy the device will deliver and in what order.

Again, the programming options for devices are extensive, but it's good to know the LRL and URL for a pacemaker and, for an ICD, the heart rates at which treatments will be given. A quick example:

Mr. Smith has an ICD that is programmed with an LRL of 60, a URL of 120, and a setting that tells it to treat fast rhythms above 200 beats per minute. If Mr. Smith were to find his heart rate well below 60 beats per minute, that would potentially be concerning, as the pacemaker portion of his device is supposed to keep his rate above 60. (It would be extremely uncommon for this to happen.) If his heart rate is between 120 and 200, it simply means that his heart is beating on its own. Finally, if his heart rate goes above 200, he should expect treatments from his ICD.

TESTING YOUR DEVICE

The first time you have your device interrogated will depend on many factors. Some patients will get their first check the day after implant, before they leave the hospital. Other patients will have their device checked while still unconscious, before leaving the operating room. Either way, it will usually be interrogated before you leave the hospital. Your first in-office check will usually come anywhere from 1 week to 3 months after your implant. No matter when your first interrogation takes place, it is nothing to be worried about. There is no pain involved, and the check can often be done in less than 30 minutes.

When it comes to making sure your device is functioning properly, there are four measurements that your caregiver will take. He or she will test your device's ability to detect your own heartbeat, the device's ability to pace your heart when needed, the status of the leads, and the battery strength. In addition to taking these measurements, your caregiver will also look at all the data that that the device collects about your heart.

THRESHOLD

For starters, your caregiver will test the **pacing threshold** of each of the wires in your system. The pacing threshold is a measurement that tells the caregiver how much energy it takes to make your heart beat. As you can imagine, if your heart required 10 volts of electricity to make it beat, but your device only has the capacity to deliver 5 volts, it could cause a real problem. This is one of the most important measurements to obtain. During the test, which can be done rapidly, some patients feel their heart race a little, but more commonly there is no sensation during the testing.

The threshold, or minimum amount of energy needed to make your heart beat, will vary slightly throughout the life of your device. Small variations in your threshold levels between device checks are fine, and if needed, your caregiver can alter the amount of energy that the device puts out to each lead. For example, if your check shows that your threshold is up to 2 volts from a previous measurement of 1 volt, your caregiver may program an output of 4 volts. Programming the extra energy is called a **safety margin.** It is simply an amount of energy above the minimum amount required to pace your heart. The safety margin is added to compensate for normal, day-to-day variations in threshold.

A higher threshold will require your caregiver to program more energy output from your device, which may have some impact on how long your battery will last. A very high threshold, defined here as any threshold that requires more energy than the device can deliver, will likely require either a new lead or another procedure to reposition the existing lead. A low threshold is not a problem and will simply make your battery last longer.

SENSING

The next thing your caregiver will check is your device's ability to recognize **(sense)** your own heartbeat. This is extremely important in all patients but is of special importance in those of you with ICDs. If your ICD were "blind" to your own heart rhythm, it would never know when to deliver a life-saving shock. **Sensing** is also important for pacemaker patients, or for the pacemaker incorporated in your ICD or CRT. If your device doesn't know if or when your own heart is beating, how will it know when to step in and help out?

In order to determine how well your device is seeing your heartbeat, your caregiver may need to slow or lower the programmed pacing rate. Although most patients feel nothing during this 5-second test, some patients may feel a little lightheaded for a few seconds.

After obtaining this measurement on each of your leads, your caregiver can adjust the settings of the device if needed. Altering the ability of the device to recognize your own heart rhythm is called programming the **sensitivity level.** This determines how sensitive your device is to electrical signals.

It is also possible that the device can be programmed to be *too* sensitive, which may result in the device seeing and counting electrical signals that aren't coming from the heart, but instead coming from some sort of outside interference. In other words, it is seeing too much. Conversely, if not programmed to be sensitive enough, the device may not see your heartbeat at all, essentially becoming "blind."

IMPEDANCE

The next critical measurement that your caregiver will assess is the electrical resistance or **impedance** level on each of your leads. This is done in a few seconds. If the impedance level on your lead(s) is within normal limits, this indicates that the lead is electrically normal. However, if your impedance level is too low, it can indicate a possible break in the covering or insulation of the lead. If too high, it can indicate either a fracture or a developing fracture in your lead's conductor wire (the wire that delivers the electricity to your heart). The treatments for these problems can vary depending on the specific situation. Commonly, if a problem is developing in the wire or the insulation, another procedure may be necessary to place a new lead.

BATTERY

Your caregiver will check your device's battery level. Although it is difficult to predict precisely how long the battery will last, generally your caregiver can give you a very good "ballpark" of when your device's battery will get to the point when it needs to be replaced.

Once your battery reaches its **elective replacement indicator,** or **ERI,** it's time for a new device. At ERI, your device has about 3 months of full usage before battery strength becomes a real concern. This allows time to schedule your procedure when convenient for you and your doctor. If for some reason you were to wait and still not have the device replaced after the 3 months, it would eventually reach a point when the battery is almost completely depleted. Unfortunately the term used for this is **end of life (EOL)**, referring to the end of the functional life of the battery. It's a term that can cause concern to the patient when they hear the caregiver talking about "end of life." When the device reaches EOL, several features of the pacemaker are turned off in order to preserve battery strength for the most important functions of the device. The features that are turned off are features not essential to keeping you alive. If you are regular with your follow-ups, your device hopefully will never reach a point where the battery is very nearly depleted without you having adequate warning that something needs to be done. However, many patients find it comforting to know that when your caregiver tells you that it's time for a "battery change," you still have several months of normal usage before getting a new battery becomes extremely urgent.

When it does come time to have your battery changed, your physician will actually replace the entire device. The battery is carefully sealed inside the pulse generator and can't be removed; therefore, getting a new battery requires getting a new device. Provided your leads are in good working condition, your doctor will simply unplug the leads from your old device and plug those existing leads into a brand new device. This allows you to have the most up-to-date technology available. Many patients ask why the manufacturers can't simply make a device with rechargeable or replaceable batteries. In fact, such a device did exist at one time, but the need to recharge the device wasn't always well accepted by patients. Also, technology moves fast, and cardiac devices are no exception. A device that never needed to be replaced would eventually lag behind newer devices with up-to-date technology.

ADVANCED FEATURES

Before completing your interrogation, your caregiver will check all the information about your heart that the device has gathered. The type of information collected can vary a great deal depending on the type of device. For example, ICDs gather extra information regarding your activity levels, and most devices can also chart the time you actually used your pacemaker, versus the time your heart spends beating on its own.

Some of the more advanced features are found in the newer CRT devices. As an example, some CRT devices can monitor for fluid retention in your lungs, which may indicate developing heart failure. All of this information can be useful to your caregivers as they decide how to best manage your heart disease. In some of today's never devices, however, the parameters monitored by the device can detect problems before you have any visible symptoms. The device can wirelessly relay this information to your caregiver, who can use that information to adjust your medications over the phone, potentially keeping you from needing a visit to the office or the emergency room, or even a hospitalization.

A BEEPING DEVICE

Some devices are designed to inform you of potential problems by making an audible noise, often some sort of beeping. Your device can alert you for a variety of problems, including major issues or minor things that require your attention, such as when your battery reaches ERI. Each device is different, so ask your caregiver what a beeping device means for you. Also, at your first check, ask your caregiver to turn on the beeper so you can hear what it sounds like. Finally, ask them what you should do if you hear it beeping. Again, in some devices, beeping would require a call to your doctor when convenient; in others, it would require a trip to the emergency room.

HOME MONITORING SYSTEMS

A home monitoring system allows you to have your device checked from home. The earliest type of remote monitoring was for pacemakers only and worked over the telephone. Using a device provided by the caregiver, patients could call into the doctor's office and send a heart tracing over the phone. This heart tracing would tell the caregiver if the battery was okay, and if the device had any major problems. Many pacemaker patients are still using this system today. It is called **trans-telephonic monitoring.** Generally, if you use trans-telephonic monitoring, you will need to call in on a regular basis. The frequency of calls will depend on the specific protocol your caregiver prefers. If everything looks good on the phone checks, then you will only need to go in to the caregiver's office for a full check about once a year.

Although this is a great system, it does have its limitations. As noted, it is only capable of giving you a very basic check—sufficient for most pacemaker patients. Some of the newer home monitoring systems, however, can generate a full interrogation of your pacemaker, ICD, or CRT device from home. Programming the device is not possible remotely.

The new systems come with a small communicator that is designed for your home (Figure 2). The communicator can be placed anywhere, but most patients put it in their bedroom. As noted earlier, your communicator may either have a wand on it or be wireless with a small antenna, depending on your device. The wireless communicators will reach out to your device in the middle of the night—every night in some cases—and check your device without you feeling anything, even while you sleep. The "wanded" communicators often have a flashing light to notify you that you need a check. When you see the flashing light, you simply place the wand over your device for about 30 seconds, and you are done.

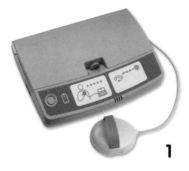
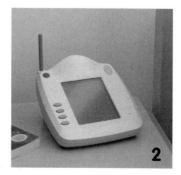
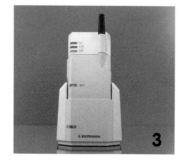
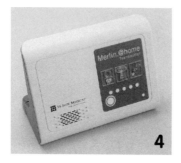

Figure 2. Examples of home monitoring systems from different device manufacturers; clockwise, from top left: (1) Medtronic CareLink; (2) Boston Scientific Latitude; (3) Biotronik Home Monitoring; (4) St. Jude Merlin Transmitter. Used with permission of Medtronic, Inc., Boston Scientific Corporation, Biotronik Inc., and St. Jude Medical.

Once your communicator gathers this information, it sends it to your caregiver through the Internet. Some communicators send this via a home phone line, others via cell phone signals. Either way, once it has been sent in, your physician can access it from anywhere in the world via an Internet connection. This allows you to get your regular follow-up done from home (Figure 3).

These communicators are also wonderful for ICD patients after a shock. Often, your caregiver will instruct you to simply send a communication after a shock instead of automatically making a trip to the emergency room or even the doctor's office. As soon as your caregiver receives and reviews this information, he/she can see exactly what happened and why you received a therapy.

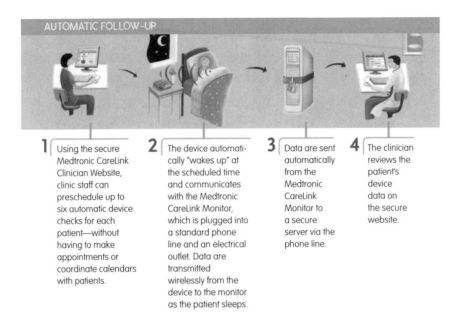

AUTOMATIC FOLLOW-UP

1 | Using the secure Medtronic CareLink Clinician Website, clinic staff can preschedule up to six automatic device checks for each patient—without having to make appointments or coordinate calendars with patients.

2 | The device automatically "wakes up" at the scheduled time and communicates with the Medtronic CareLink Monitor, which is plugged into a standard phone line and an electrical outlet. Data are transmitted wirelessly from the device to the monitor as the patient sleeps.

3 | Data are sent automatically from the Medtronic CareLink Monitor to a secure server via the phone line.

4 | The clinician reviews the patient's device data on the secure website.

Figure 3. Transmission of information from a home monitoring system. Some differences exist between different systems of different companies. Used with permission of Medtronic, Inc.

Most patients who begin using the remote monitoring system like it very much and appreciate the peace of mind they receive from knowing they have a link directly to the caregiver. They can be monitored daily from home, something that wasn't possible just a few years ago, and can follow up at their doctor's office when needed. Talk to your caregiver about home monitoring so that the two of you can decide the best and most comfortable way to obtain follow-up for your device.

Chapter 7

Possible Complications

If you or a loved one is preparing for surgery, it is natural to have some anticipation beforehand because any invasive procedure carries the risk of potential complications. The good news about cardiac devices is that after the initial implant, the long-term risks are quite low. The physician or nurse who first talks to you about your need for a device should talk to you about possible complications of the surgery. If they do not bring it up, make sure you ask. Specifically, you should ask about the risks of having the device implanted, how often those risks occur, and whether there are any problems or complications that could be expected later. This information will help you know what to expect before, during, and after the surgery.

COMPLICATIONS OF DEVICE IMPLANT DIRECTLY RELATED TO THE PROCEDURE

There are a variety of potential problems that could occur with device implant, but many of them are very unlikely. In fact, the vast majority of device procedures happen with virtually no complications. It is much like listening to an advertisement on television for a medication in which you hear a large number of potential side effects listed, most of which you never think twice about. However, the following major potential complications should be explained by the caregiver describing the implant procedure.

Lead Dislodgement

Lead dislodgement is one of the most common post-implant complications. Although the leads are secured into place at the initial implant, they can still dislodge or fall out of position. The leads that are placed in your heart eventually must become scarred into place. It is the scar tissue (also called fibrosis) around the leads that really holds them in place for the long term. The leads do have a specific mechanism at the tip of the lead that helps to anchor them in place initially, before the scar tissue forms. Most commonly, the lead has a tiny screw that actually screws into the inside of the heart to hold the lead in place. This screw is very small, so there is no concern that it will damage the heart tissue. The use of a screw is called **active fixation.** Another mechanism commonly used to hold leads in place is small tines that look like a grappling hook, although they are very soft. These tines may be better for securing the lead when it needs to be placed in the vein at a particular angle (Figure 1). This mechanism is called **passive fixation.**

It takes about 6 weeks for your body to form the scar tissue or fibrosis around the leads. Therefore, the chances of a lead dislodging are highest within the first 6 weeks following lead placement. Rates of lead dislodgement vary by hospital, but on average, only 1 to 3 out of every 100 patients will experience this issue. If the lead moves or dislodges, it will likely require another operation to reposition the lead(s) so that it is functioning

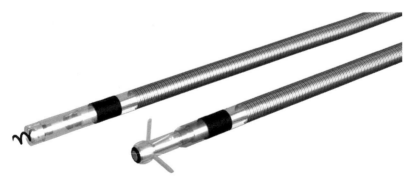

Figure 1. Side-by-side of an active fixation and a passive fixation lead. Used with permission of Medtronic, Inc.

normally. Figure 2 shows x-rays of correct pacemaker lead placement and a dislodged pacemaker lead. Your doctor may perform several different tests to determine whether the leads have indeed dislodged. A few of the most helpful are a simple ECG, x-ray, and/or device interrogation with the programmer. All of these tests are usually done before you leave the hospital following device implant.

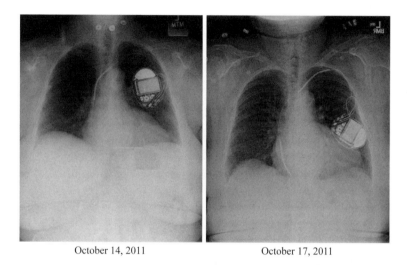

October 14, 2011   October 17, 2011

Figure 2. (Left) Ventricular lead in the right ventricle in an appropriate position. (Right) Ventricular lead that has dislodged or moved in the same patient a few days later.

This risk of dislodgement is the reason your activities may be somewhat limited for the first several weeks after an implant. However, once this initial period passes, the risk of dislodgement is incredibly small. In fact, after the scar tissue has formed around the leads, they can be difficult to remove.

Collapsed Lung (Pneumothorax)

The leads are generally placed in a large vein just below your clavicle. This vein is located close to the top portion of your lung. It is possible that during the insertion of the device, the lung could be punctured by either the needle or the wire as the lead is being placed. The risk of having a collapsed lung, the medical term for which is **pneumothorax** *(noom-o-thor-ax)*, is less than 1 in 100 procedures. However, it is a known complication, and it can occur. Therefore, you should be informed about this possibility.

If this issue does occur, the treatment depends on how severe the pneumothorax is. For example, if only a small portion of the upper lung collapses, it may not be necessary for your caregivers to do anything but to observe, as it is possible that your body will expand the small collapsed portion on its own. If a large portion of the lung collapses, the lung would have to be re-expanded by having another procedure to insert a **chest tube** in the side of your chest. In either case, the time that you need to be in the hospital following the procedure would be extended by at least a couple of days. The good news is that there should be no long-term issues resulting from this surgical complication, should it occur.

Infection

Any time you undergo a procedure where the skin is opened, regardless of how careful the caregivers are to maintain everything in a sterile, germ-free environment, there is always a risk of infection (Figure 3). The risk of infection varies a great deal from institution to institution. Ideally, an institution has an infection rate of 1 in 200 patients or less.

The most common signs of an infection would be redness, soreness, and/or warmth of the skin over the device; an opening of the incision; or draining from the incision. Seeing any portion of the device or lead coming through the skin is also considered a sign of infection, even if there are no other symptoms. Any of these signs or symptoms should be reported to your pacemaker caregiver. An infection may occur very soon after the implant or very late, even years later. It all depends on the type of infection and the type of bacteria or organism that is causing the infection.

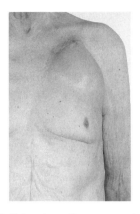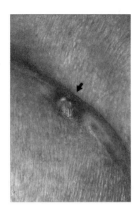

Figure 3. (Left) A patient with a very prominent area after device implantation. This patient had a collection of blood (called a hematoma) that formed after the procedure. When a collection of blood such as this occurs, it can put the patient at a higher risk of an infection, which this patient subsequently developed. (Right) A photograph taken some time after a device was implanted. The arrow points to an area where a portion of the device is eroding or wearing through the skin.

Although an infection is usually not the result of anything you have done, it is still important to follow instructions closely after implant. You should be told to avoid touching the incision early after the procedure, and it's probably best to avoid putting any creams or ointments on the incision site. Until it has healed well, avoid submerging your incision in water, even a bath, and certainly you should avoid immersing it in public swimming pools or hot tubs.

If the location of your device becomes infected, it will likely require removal of the device and leads to allow a full healing to take place. Some small infections only affect the pocket or location of the device, without causing infection in the bloodstream. However, it is possible that bacteria on one of the leads could infect your bloodstream. In this case, the device site itself may or may not become infected as well. Regardless, once there is *any* infection, it generally means that the entire implanted system must be removed until the infection has completely resolved. Once the infection is gone, your physician can re-implant your device and leads. The process of removing a system is called **extraction,** which is discussed below.

Perforation of the Heart Wall

One of the most severe surgical complications is fortunately one of the most rare as well. It is commonly known as perforation. Perforation can happen as the leads are put in position or as the small lead screw is extended into the heart muscle. During lead placement, it is possible that the wall of the heart could be punctured. If the wall of the heart is punctured, and blood begins to surround the sac around the heart, also called the **pericardium** (*pair-a-card-e-um*), significant problems can occur. If enough blood collects in the sac around the heart, it can prevent the heart from functioning normally. Therefore, the blood needs to be removed as quickly as possible. Usually the blood is removed with a small needle or a catheter. Very rarely, surgery may be required to correct a collection of blood in the sac around the heart, especially if there has been a sizable tear in the heart muscle. The chance of needing surgery is very low. It is so uncommon, in fact, that it is difficult to accurately state how often this happens. A close estimate is about 2 in 1,000 cases. The likelihood of this occurring is probably slightly greater in women than in men because of differences in anatomy.

It's also possible, although again very unlikely, that the tip of the lead or the tip of the screw might barely extend beyond the wall of the heart, not enough that any bleeding occurs, but enough that the sac around the heart can be irritated and inflamed. This is called **pericarditis** and can result in chest pain and a variety of associated symptoms. This problem will sometimes subside spontaneously, but other times will require treatment. Some patients will respond to anti-inflammatory agents like ibuprofen; very rarely, it may require that the lead be moved.

Complications Related to Anesthesia

Any surgical procedure can have complications related to anesthetic drugs being given to you. It's reasonable for you to ask the doctor doing the procedure if there are possible complications of the anesthetic drugs that you should be told about. However, risk of complications related to anesthesia for placement of a cardiac device is very low because most procedures, with the exception of extraction (removal) of pacing leads, do not require being put completely to sleep using a **general anesthetic.** Instead, you are given medications in your vein that simply make you very sleepy, but do not render you unconscious. Even so, most patients do sleep through the procedure and usually have no memory of what took place.

OTHER QUESTIONS REGARDING COMPLICATIONS AT THE TIME OF IMPLANT

Can placement of a device result in heart attack, stroke, or death? Obviously, these are major events that you would want to know about. The simple answer is, it's possible, but such complications almost never occur. The device is placed on the right side of the heart, which is not the side of the circulation that connects to the brain. Therefore, the chance of having a stroke is very small or almost nonexistent.

Likewise, the risk of death is extremely small. It is possible that if the heart wall was torn and there was major bleeding, as discussed earlier, this complication could result in death or brain damage if not corrected quickly enough. However, damage to the heart wall during a procedure is very uncommon, and once recognized, the doctor doing the implant would act quickly to manage the situation.

It would also be very uncommon for you to have a heart attack. If you know that you have coronary disease, and especially if you have ongoing chest pain or angina, then the caregiver seeing you prior to the procedure will probably want to evaluate the status of your coronary disease before moving forward with the implant procedure. This is to ensure that you will tolerate the sedation you are given during a procedure.

LATER COMPLICATIONS

There are other problems that can potentially affect patients at any time following device implant. Although rare, the problems described below do occur. Hopefully, learning more about these potential complications helps you understand why it is so important to have your device closely monitored by your healthcare team.

Unacceptable Function of the Lead

Dislodgement

As mentioned above, it is possible that a lead could move or dislodge from your heart. If dislodgement occurs, the lead may not be capable of stimulating your heart or sensing your heart's electrical activity as it should. Although a chest x-ray may help your doctor determine that a lead has dislodged, some dislodgements are not detected this way. Perhaps the lead has moved such a tiny amount that it cannot be seen on the x-ray, or perhaps there has been a lot of scar tissue formed at the tip of the lead that is causing problems with the way it functions. Regardless, if the lead is functioning very poorly and it is taking too much energy to stimulate your heart, or it is not able to stimulate the heart at all (a problem called **failure to capture**), it may be necessary for you to undergo another procedure to move the lead or put in a different lead.

Fracture or Insulation Problem

As the lead ages, like any product, it can wear out. An implanted lead could develop damage to the insulation material that coats the wire(s), or a wire itself might break. If either of these problems develops, a new lead would need to be placed. If you are being followed on a regular basis, either through a home monitoring system or directly in your doctor's office, the device clinic will often have clues that a problem is developing with the lead before there is an actual change in how it functions. This is one of the reasons it is so important to be regularly checked by a device clinic.

Stimulation of Your Diaphragm or Muscles

Your device uses small electrical impulses to stimulate your heart muscle. In some rare instances, these small electrical impulses can also stimulate other muscles in your torso. To make sure this doesn't happen, when the doctor places the leads, they are also tested to be certain that they stimulate nothing other than your heart muscle. More specifically, the doctor wants to make sure that the leads are not stimulating your **diaphragm,** the major muscle separating your abdomen and your chest that moves up and down when you breathe, or any other muscles in your torso. However, even if the operating room testing is normal, once you are out of surgery and upright or moving around it is possible that the position of the lead could shift slightly, resulting in such stimulation. If this does happen, it is not dangerous, just very bothersome. It may be similar to having severe hiccups where you feel a jerking sensation. Again, it is not dangerous to you, and it doesn't harm the device or the leads, but it can be a real nuisance and can certainly affect your quality of life. If that happens, you should let your caregivers know. It may be possible that they can adjust the energy output on the device to avoid this unwanted stimulation yet still be able to stimulate your heart muscle as needed. In some cases, surgery may be needed to move the lead to a new position.

Pain

It's expected that you will have some discomfort immediately after the pro-cedure at the site where the device has been placed. Most patients report that this only lasts a few days, and your caregivers will send you home with pain medications to use as needed. (More information on follow-up is included in Chapter 6.)

A small number of patients may experience discomfort at the site of the device (the **pocket**). This discomfort is different from the acute surgical discomfort in that it can show up after the initial healing has taken place. The cause of this "pocket pain" is usually difficult to determine. If the pain is occurring in the early weeks or months after implant, it may be worth a period of observation to see if it goes away. It's possible that as additional fibrotic material (scar tissue) forms around the device, the discomfort may stop. If it persists, then it sometimes requires another procedure to revise the pocket. You have learned about the possible risks of surgery, so it is understandable that your physician may take a "wait and see" approach to pain at the pocket. Sometimes, because patients feel uncomfortable with the new machinery in their body, they may interpret their discomfort and negative feelings as pain. For many patients, once they learn to accept the device as a good and necessary treatment, their pain and discomfort go away. Many patients report that they eventually don't even notice their device anymore because it feels like a part of their body. Regardless of the cause, it is important to let your caregivers know if you are experiencing pocket pain so that they can manage it effectively.

Erosion

If the device has been placed too close to the skin or if you lose a lot of weight following the procedure, it's possible that the device or a portion of a lead could erode or work its way through the skin. If you notice any part of the system that seems very prominent or poking out, or seems to alter the appearance of the skin, you should draw it to the attention of your caregivers (Figure 4). If the caregiver believes that there is the potential for erosion of the system, they will want to react before it actually occurs. Once there is a true breach of the skin, by definition the system is infected, and the entire system would probably need to be removed.

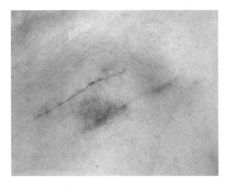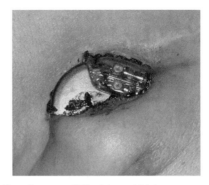

Figure 4. (Left) A patient after a pacemaker implant. There is some mild bruising, which is common. However, there is no redness or any signs of infection. (Right) This pacemaker has completed eroded through the skin.

COMPLICATIONS UNIQUE TO ICDS

Inappropriate Shocks

ICDs are very sophisticated devices. The computer chip that runs the device maintains a constant surveillance of your heart rhythm. The ICD is designed to shock or pace your heart when it determines that your heart has reached a certain fast rate, determined by your doctor.

A normal fast rate is one that everyone experiences when exercising. It is called **sinus tachycardia.** Another fast rate that is not normal, but also not life-threatening, is called **atrial tachycardia.** The ICD isn't intended to treat these rhythms. Abnormal, life-threatening, fast heart rates called **ventricular tachycardia** or **ventricular fibrillation** are the rhythms your defibrillator is intended to treat. The device has to be smart enough to distinguish between different fast rhythms. Although ICDs are very sophisticated and improve with each new device made by manufacturers, they are not perfect and aren't always able to distinguish between different rhythms. In fact, about 20% of patients with an ICD will receive a shock when they don't require one. When you receive a shock for one of the two fast heart rates that the ICD is not designed to treat, it is called an **inappropriate shock.** It is inappropriate because we only want to shock life-threatening fast heart rates. Although inappropriate shocks may be unpleasant and burdensome, they often occur because devices are designed to err on the side of caution. In other words, if the device thinks you may be having a dangerous arrhythmia, but is not 100% sure, it will deliver a shock anyway. This is to ensure that life-saving therapy is not withheld when it should be delivered. As ICD technology continues to improve, the chances of receiving an inappropriate shock are decreasing.

In general, an inappropriate shock is not life-threatening. The worst-case scenario would be that your heart is shocked when it isn't necessary, and that the shock itself causes ventricular tachycardia or ventricular fibrillation. However, if that happens, your device should once again detect the bad heart rhythm, and a second shock would be delivered, restoring a normal heart rhythm.

In most patients, the only problem is simply that they experience a shock. This isn't much of a concern to your doctor, from a medical standpoint, but may be of concern to you. If your heart is truly going very fast in one of the potentially dangerous rhythms, ventricular tachycardia or ventricular fibrillation, you will most likely be passing out or will have already passed out before the shock is delivered. If you are not fully awake when the shock is delivered, you may not even remember it. However, if you receive an inappropriate shock when you are wide awake, you will almost certainly feel the shock, which most patients describe as being unpleasant.

People describe a shock in a variety of ways. Some describe it as having been kicked in the chest, while others describe it as accidentally grabbing hold of a live electrical socket. We have also heard patients in rural areas describe it as feeling similar to accidentally touching an electric fence. The good news is that the shock lasts less than a second and is over before you even know what happened. (For more information, see Chapter 8.)

You should also understand that many fast, even potentially dangerous heart rhythms might be detected and treated by rapid pacing from the ICD. If the rhythm responds to the rapid pacing, you may not require a shock. The term for this is **antitachycardia pacing (ATP),** and almost all ICD patients should have this particular feature turned on. Patients do not usually have any symptoms associated with receiving ATP, and often do not even know that this therapy was delivered. They may, however, be aware that their heart is going fast prior to this special type of pacing therapy, but they don't feel the pacing itself, nor is there any shock delivered. ATP has eliminated many shocks for patients, both appropriate and inappropriate. In fact, it could be the most patient-friendly feature ever developed for the ICD.

What you are told to do if you receive a shock will likely vary depending on the preference of your caregivers. Many caregivers will suggest that if you receive a shock and you feel fine after the shock, that you notify them during normal business hours if at all possible. If you are on a remote monitoring system, they may have additional information transmitted to them so that they can review the actual heart tracing that occurred when you had the shock. Other caregivers may prefer that you go to the emergency room if you have a shock. However, most medical professionals would agree that if you are not feeling well after a shock, you will probably need to be seen somewhat urgently, and you should strongly consider going to the emergency room or calling 911. **Do *not* drive yourself to the hospital!**

Multiple Shocks

At times, the ICD may deliver multiple shocks. This may be because there are recurrent bad heart rhythms, which all require treatment to keep you alive. However, if they are occurring very frequently, you should go to the emergency room as directed by your caregiver. (Different caregivers will have different opinions about what "very frequent" shocks really means. Certainly more than three shocks within 24 hours would fit this definition.)

We normally find that in this instance, patients are quite eager to get to the ER to stop the incessant shocking.

Multiple shocks can be delivered for inappropriate reasons as well. As we discussed earlier, your device may shock you for a fast, abnormal heart rate coming from the top chambers of the heart. (The most common of these is called **atrial fibrillation.**) One reason you may receive multiple shocks for this problem is that the device isn't specifically designed to treat fast rhythms occurring in the atria—it's designed for fast rhythms coming from the ventricles. When a shock doesn't slow down your heart or correct the abnormal rhythm, the device will keep recognizing the fast rhythm and continue trying to stop it, leading to multiple shocks.

Whatever the cause of multiple shocks, whether they are appropriate or inappropriate, you should be evaluated if this happens. Notify your caregiver or follow whatever process they have already explained to you, and go to the appropriate office or emergency room. If you are experiencing multiple shocks, you should not attempt to drive yourself to seek medical attention. Most likely you will need to call an ambulance or paramedic service if multiple shocks are being delivered.

Therapies Accidentally Turned Off

It is important that your ICD always have the ability to deliver pacing treatment or shocks when needed. It is possible that if a caregiver is programming your device, therapies could be turned off, either for a specific reason or accidentally, and not turned back on. The most likely scenario would be that your therapies were turned off for some surgical procedure during which you were monitored for any abnormal heart rhythms, and then after the surgery, the caregivers failed to reactivate the therapies. It's obviously not good to go home with an ICD that is turned off, but it isn't as big of an issue since home monitoring systems have been developed. These systems should spot the problem and send a message to your caregiver that the therapies are not turned on as they should be. Not to worry though—most caregivers are extremely cautious about checking and double-checking that therapies are turned on and appropriately set at the end of any programming session. Going home with a device that is turned off is very rare.

Extractions

As noted above, an infection may sometimes require that your device and leads be removed. This is called an **extraction.** Infection is not the only reason for extraction, but it is certainly the most common cause. Other reasons for extraction would include the need to place a new or different lead when there isn't enough room in the blood vessel to allow another lead to be placed—that is, one lead must be removed in order to get another one in. At times, children who receive an implant will literally outgrow the leads, and in these cases, the leads need to be extracted. Generally speaking, the younger you are when you receive your first device, the greater the chance that you may need an extraction at some point in your future.

Because an extraction is a very specialized procedure, there are additional things that should be discussed with your caregiver and questions you should be prepared to ask.

1. What complications should I know about?
2. How often do the complications occur?
3. Could I die as a result of the procedure?
4. Are there any alternatives to an extraction?
5. How much experience do you and your team have doing extractions?
6. Do you use laser equipment to remove the leads?

Because the leads have scar tissue around them, and because that scar tissue tends to increase the longer the leads are in place, they can be very difficult to remove. This means that the leads, which are connected to your heart or to the major blood vessels, have to be peeled away from those structures without damage to your heart or blood vessels. The main concern is that, in an attempt to remove the leads, the heart or blood vessels could be torn. A significant tear could be sudden and, if large enough, could result in excess blood loss and possibly death. For all these reasons, lead extraction is not a procedure to be taken lightly.

Extraction should be performed by individuals who have significant experience with this procedure, and you should specifically ask your doctor about his or her level of experience. Many doctors will actually refer patients to other large centers for this particular procedure. At this time, extractions are generally done with a laser. The laser helps to literally cut through the scar tissue. It does so in a very precise way to try to avoid damage to the heart or blood vessels.

Even in the most experienced hands, there are risks of major complications or even death with an extraction procedure. It is difficult to determine the exact risks, because many institutions still quote older numbers that were determined before laser extraction became available, when extraction methods were much cruder. At that time, the risk of a potentially life-threatening complication from an extraction was about 2 out of 100, and the risk of death was slightly less than 1 in 100. These risks are probably even lower when the procedure is performed by an experienced physician using a laser system today, but extraction still may carry significant risk.

Again, if your caregiver tells you that you need an extraction, you should be prepared to ask about the amount of experience the institution has doing extractions, the risks posed from an extraction, the specific types of risks, the rate of risks associated with an extraction, and the type of equipment they would be using.

Chapter 8

The Shocking Truth

Your knowledge of defibrillator shocks may be based on what you have seen on television. You have likely seen TV shows with people getting shocked from the "paddles" (also called an **external defibrillator**) who then proceed to "bounce" from the large jolt. If you are like most ICD patients, you may have skipped right to this chapter, wondering if this portrayal of a shock is accurate. A lot of patients wonder if implantable defibrillators have the same jarring effect, or if it's simply TV hype.

If you did skip right to this chapter, don't worry—you are not alone in your curiosity about shocks. If there is one thing that many ICD patients seem to have in common, it is some level of preoccupation about getting shocked. For the most part, people who have never been shocked want to know everything there is to know about the shock—most importantly, what it will feel like. Those of you who have been shocked may be reading this chapter to see if there are any secrets to making the experience a bit easier. Although reading this chapter won't necessarily make your next shock experience pleasant, our hope is that the knowledge you gain here will bring you peace of mind and less discomfort.

WHAT DOES A SHOCK FEEL LIKE?

People describe shocks in many different ways. Some say it feels like a kick to the chest, others compare it to a jolt from an electric fence, and so on. Patient surveys have revealed that on a pain scale ranging from 1 to 10, with 1 representing "no pain" and 10 representing "worst pain imaginable," most patients rate an ICD shock as a 6. Most patients also say that the shock is more sudden and frightening than it is painful.[1, 2]

Although most ICD patients would agree with these analogies and ratings, at best they are a bit incomplete, and at worst, perhaps a bit misleading for many reasons. For starters, if you spend time talking to patients who have had many shocks over the years, they will tell you that each one was its own unique experience. Recent research suggests that patients may remember a shock as less painful if they know that it was delivered to stop a life-threatening arrhythmia.[3] In other words, the shock was appropriate. If you've read Chapter 7, you know it is possible for the ICD to be "tricked" into thinking that your heart needs a shock when it actually doesn't, thus resulting in an inappropriate shock. Some research suggests that patients may remember inappropriate shocks as more painful than appropriate shocks. Perhaps the knowledge that the ICD saved a patient's life makes him or her more accepting of the shock experience. There are multiple other factors that will affect how the shock actually feels: everything from the positioning of your body to your state of mind during the shock. To better understand this, let's first look at what a shock actually is, and what it is that you are feeling.

[1] Pelletier D, Gallagher R, Mitten-Lewis S, McKinley S, & Squire J. Australian implantable cardiac defibrillator recipients: Quality-of-life issues. *Int J Nursing Pract*, 2002; 8: 68–74.

[2] Ahmad M, Bloomstein L, Roelke M, Bernstein AD, & Parsonnet V. Patients' attitudes toward implanted defibrillator shocks. *Pacing and Clinical Electrophysiology*, 2000; 23: 934–938.

[3] Marcus G, Chan D, & Redberg R. Recollection of pain due to inappropriate versus appropriate implantable cardioverter-defibrillator shocks. *Pacing and Clinical Electrophysiology*, March 2011; 34: 348–353.

WHAT IS A SHOCK?

Just the thought of a shock may frighten you, especially if you think of a shock as a jolt of electricity coursing through your body. Fear not, because this is not an accurate description of what happens during a shock or what you will feel. In fact, you won't actually "feel" the electricity at all! What you will feel is your body's response to the electricity—that is, the muscles in your chest, back, and stomach suddenly contract. This sudden, hard contraction of your muscles causes your body to jolt or jerk very quickly and intensely. This jerk is what you actually feel.

It would be reasonable to ask, "Why not just turn down the electricity so my muscles don't jerk so hard?" When your heart is in a potentially dangerous rhythm coming from the bottom chambers of the heart, that is, ventricular fibrillation or ventricular tachycardia, the most effective way (and sometimes the only way) to get it back to normal is to apply enough electricity to the heart, and in so doing to the rest of your body, to reset or reorganize the heart's rhythm. The sudden contraction of the heart muscle as a result of the shock causes it to pause, allowing it to return to a normal rhythm. The good news is, by the time you realize what happened, the shock is over and done. It may be helpful to reflect on the shock as a life-saving event as opposed to a negative experience.

When you think of a shock experience as the contraction of several major muscles, you may better understand why relaxation can help manage shock pain. Research shows that patients who can relax their muscles before a shock is delivered may perceive the shock as less painful than patients who are tense when they are shocked. In fact, psychologists recommend that after receiving a shock, you may benefit from lying or sitting down and trying to relax all of your muscles. This will help you remain calm and may also make any subsequent shocks feel less painful. Relaxation can involve taking several deep breaths or visualizing a place that makes you feel peaceful. Relaxation may also include repeating positive phrases such as "I know my ICD is keeping me safe" or "Everything is going to be okay." Of course, this may be easier said than done when you have just had an event. It will take a great deal of effort on your part to stay calm, but having this reaction plan in place can help. As described by the patient scenario below, your physical and mental state during a shock can make a big difference in your emotional outcome.

FEELING OF THE MIND

There is no other factor that will affect what a shock feels like more than your state of mind. To illustrate this point, here is a story from a patient who has had his ICD almost 20 years.

> I had two shocks a few years apart that were completely different. I mean, everything was the same with the ICD and the settings and all that stuff, but the circumstances surrounding them couldn't have been more different. For the first shock, I just happened to be wearing a heart monitor that displays your heart rate when I felt my heart start to race. I lay down and immediately looked at the monitor to see the rate rising rapidly. I knew my ICD was programmed to shock me when it got to 200, so as the monitor approached 200 within seconds, I held my breath and waited. I was panicked . . . but nothing happened. Then I really panicked. I went from being afraid that I was going to get a shock to being afraid that I *wasn't* going to get a shock. I was afraid I was going to die; my device wasn't going to work! My thoughts were racing, and I was scared out of my mind when the shock finally hit me. It had only been a total of about 15 seconds, but it felt like an eternity. When the shock finally did come, I must have jumped a mile off the bed when it hit me. It was horrible. This sure was no shock from an electric fence. It was much worse than that. It was one of the worst experiences of my life. In fact, I was miserable for the next year of my life . . . always waiting for another unpleasant event to happen.

> Fast-forward several years to another shock. Working in the medical field, I had the opportunity to attend a medical conference that was full of cardiologists. While I was there, I felt my heart start racing again . . . just like before. I alerted my co-worker, and within seconds, several cardiologists surrounded me. They laid me down, took my pulse, called 911, and had a programmer for my device on its way in the seconds before I got shocked. I was in good hands, and I knew it. Over the next 5 minutes or so, I actually got three shocks—all the while knowing I was in good hands and I was going to be okay. Sure, I was still nervous, and I still felt the shocks, but it was nothing like the first experience. I was mentally calm, relaxed, and prepared. It really wasn't bad at all. In fact, it didn't make for a bad year—it really only ruined my night.

We don't often hear people talk about the night that their lives were saved as a "ruined night," but it happens with ICDs. Perhaps the best thing you can do as an ICD patient who has had a shock experience is to remind yourself that you are alive because of this device. In other words, your device has given you extra time in this life, and using that time to complain about your device will only make your next shock experience worse, not better. Sometimes all it takes is a little perspective to turn a would-be bad year into only a ruined night, and a ruined night into a tough 3 minutes.

PHANTOM SHOCKS

Some of the worst-feeling shocks are shocks that you never actually receive. A **phantom shock** is when an ICD patient has a strong and certain feeling that they have been shocked, when in fact they have not. Simply put, it's your mind playing tricks on you. Nothing illustrates the power of the mind better than phantom shocks. In fact, patients who have had phantom shocks will absolutely insist that they've been shocked, describing it as feeling exactly like an actual shock. Some will even argue with their clinician after a device interrogation, insisting that the computer must be wrong, because they *felt* a shock! In a way, they are right because even though the device didn't actually shock them, they did perceive a sensation exactly like a shock. The mind is that powerful.

Phantom shocks are most common just as you are drifting off to sleep, but they can happen when sleeping or even wide awake. The most common scenario can be easily described. Remember drifting off to sleep before you got your ICD? Sometimes you would find yourself jerking awake just as you were slipping into a deep sleep. You probably thought nothing of it, rolled over, and fell asleep. Well, if that same thing happens when you're subconsciously concerned about a shock, your mind may magnify this little "jerk" and cause you to nearly jump out of bed, leaving you convinced that you've just been shocked. The mind actually magnifies this simple, normal feeling and mimics a shock.

Phantom shocks can occur in patients who have had multiple shocks and are worried about more, or even in patients who have never been shocked. Either way, if you think you've been shocked, you should seek medical attention. Do not feel embarrassed if it turns out the shock was "all in your head." Phantom shocks are fairly common and can cause physical responses just as strong as actual shocks, if not more so. The anticipation and worry that you feel when you think you have been shocked is real, even if the shock was not. Do not get discouraged or anxious if you experience one, or several, phantom shocks. Pay attention to when the phantom shocks are occurring, and what is happening in your mind and body at these times. Perhaps you are more anxious than usual because you are preoccupied with the thought of being shocked. Perhaps you are having symptoms from your heart disease, other health conditions, or concern about your family or job that are causing you to worry about your well-being. Maybe you are going through a particularly stressful time and are not taking time to relax and nurture yourself. All of these factors may result in a heightened bodily awareness that could make a phantom shock more likely.

If you are struggling with multiple phantom shock experiences, remember that you are not alone in this situation. If you have access to an ICD patient support group, you may benefit from talking with other people with ICDs. Chances are that someone else at the support group has also experienced a phantom shock. Instead of becoming frustrated with yourself, focus your energy on factors you can control.

Sometimes patients with phantom shocks are simply afraid of the un-knowns surrounding a shock situation. Making a **shock plan** with your family may decrease some of those fears (see Chapter 9 for more on shock plans). Remember to focus on the positives of the situation. Although having a phantom shock can be a confusing experience, appreciate the fact that your ICD did not need to deliver a shock because your heart rhythm is being well managed. Rest assured that your ICD is prepared to deliver a life-saving shock if you ever need one. Finally, pay attention to your stress and anxiety levels and talk to your healthcare team if you feel you could use some help with stress management.

In the passage below, Matt shares his personal experience with phantom shocks. Although this story is not representative of most patients' experiences, it will give you a sense of how emotional a phantom shock event can be.

MATT'S STORY:

I woke up in the middle of the night to what felt like a shock. Sitting up as quickly as possible and gasping for a big breath of air, I grabbed my chest. Although I was pretty sure I had been shocked, unlike almost any other ICD patient, because of my work, I had a way to check to see if I really had been shocked. Lo and behold, I had not received a real shock. Mentally, this really got to me. I thought about calling the doctors or 911, but decided to do neither.

My doctors had told me that if your device goes off once and you feel okay afterward, you can wait until morning to call and talk to the doctors. That is exactly where I found myself, and I knew that no one at the hospital at 2:00 A.M. would have any answers as to why this was happening anyway. I tried to figure it out but couldn't. Basically, my mind just raced to anything and everything . . . the good and the bad.

I thought about calling some family, as I lived alone, but realized they couldn't do anything either. Tonight I was on my own.

After about an hour of wrestling with my thoughts as I paced around, I again convinced myself that there was nothing I could do. I couldn't prevent a life-threatening heart rhythm if it was going to happen again, so I might as well try to go back to sleep. That would be the easiest way to get through the night. I got in bed and tried to pray myself to sleep. I was drifting off much faster than I had expected when my body jerked awake. Once again I was wide awake and sitting up.

I immediately realized my heart was racing but none of the other signs of a real shock where there. I had felt a shock, but again, I hadn't gotten shocked. I took a deep breath and fell backward onto my pillow. I would just have to try to sleep again.

As time passed, conscious of every heartbeat, I eventually managed to start to relax again and again, and as I was on the verge of sleep, I experienced another phantom shock. It was like having a terrible nightmare every time.

I finally relaxed but never got back to sleep. After another hour or so, I was so mentally and physically exhausted that I couldn't take it anymore. At least that's what I told God. Thankfully, He would give me the opportunity to prove myself wrong.

I went into the living room to my favorite chair. Maybe that would work. It didn't. After more time passed, I found myself lying flat on the floor staring at the television almost in a trance, hoping to trick myself into sleep. I watched television for as long as I could and finally fell asleep. Just as I was drifting off, it happened again. I must have had six or seven phantom shocks by that point, each one feeling as real as any of the real shocks that I had received in the past. I was tired and sick of fighting my own thoughts. I wondered if I would ever sleep again. I felt like I was at the end of my rope, but I didn't know what to do. There was nothing I could do.

That night turned out to be the longest of my life. I spent the entire night wrestling with my thoughts, trying to get some control over them. I tried to convince myself that I wasn't worried or scared. I tried to tell my subconscious not to worry. I tried to get some sleep, but I couldn't. I experienced 5 hours of hell like I'd never known. I had dealt with some long nights with some serious physical pain, but nothing like this. I was begging to be in the middle of one of those nights as dawn approached.

I finally decided that I wouldn't be able to sleep, so not having anything else to do and wanting to occupy my mind, I got dressed and went to work. I am not a morning person, so I am never up before the sun, but as I got dressed this morning, it was still dark. I got in the car and headed out, counting the hours until I could reach my electrophysiologist at the hospital.

I got just a few miles down the road when I was stopped at a red light on a freeway overpass. I had sat at this light hundreds of times before, looking out over the array of fast food joints and car dealerships. As I looked down the road, I noticed the horizon. Way off in the distance was the beauty of a few trees, as the road seemed to go on forever. As I sat at that light for what seemed like 10 minutes, the sun started to come up over the end of that road, up over the trees. The timing was precise as the tip of the sun edged its way above the trees just as I was pulling to a stop. I sat there and watched that sunrise, totally amazed, as if I'd never seen a glowing sun with a velvety orange sky behind it. It was the most beautiful thing I'd ever seen.

It may not sound like it, but I look back on that night with fondness. In the years before that night, I had been avoiding dealing with the mental issues that my ICD brought. That night, however, forced me to tackle them head on. Apparently I did just that, because in the 10 years since, I haven't had a single phantom shock. I've come to peace with my ICD.

CAN I PREVENT A SHOCK?

For the most part, there really isn't anything that you can do to either bring on a shock or prevent one. Taking certain drugs, especially illicit ones, or participating in activities that your cardiologist has told you your heart can't handle could increase your risk of getting a shock. However, for the most part, there really is no way of predicting when your heart may require a shock. If we could always predict that a dangerous rhythm was coming, you might not need the ICD. Your ICD simply waits for you to have one of these rhythms and then attempts to quickly correct the problem with fast pacing or a shock. Researchers are learning more and more about what causes these life-threatening rhythms, and how to prevent them, but as of now, the ICD is the best way to keep you safe. However, there are other therapies that may decrease the risk of a dangerous heart rhythm.

MEDICINES

Before ICDs were available, the only medical options were medicines called **antiarrhythmics.** These medicines are designed to prevent or decrease VT and VF. The problem, however, is that sometimes they work, but other times they do not. Taking these drugs may occasionally result in these rhythms occurring more often. Any drug can also have side effects, and those need to be discussed with the caregiver giving you the prescription.

If your electrophysiologist recommends the use of an antiarrhythmic medicine to help prevent or reduce shocks, it is important that you take your medications exactly as your doctor prescribes. Your doctor also needs to be aware of all other medications you are currently taking. Sometimes certain medications should not be taken with others, so it is important to make your healthcare team aware of all your prescriptions.

ATP

Another treatment that may help prevent shocks is **antitachycardia pacing,** or **ATP.** Again, ATP does not cure VT or VF; it is simply another type of treatment that the ICD can deliver to stop an arrhythmia. For ATP, the ICD is programmed to deliver very fast pacing pulses to your heart in an attempt to stop the fast heart rhythm. Most patients do not experience any symptoms with ATP. In fact, many patients will have no idea that they were even experiencing an arrhythmia or that any treatment was delivered. That is why ATP is sometimes referred to as "painless therapy." For many patients, the device will first deliver ATP in an attempt to break the rhythm before a shock is used.

It should be reassuring for you to know that your ICD can deliver a painless, and very often successful, therapy like ATP. The medical community acknowledges that getting shocked by the ICD is an unpleasant experience. Therefore, great efforts are being made to ensure that ICD patients only get a shock if they truly need it for a life-threatening arrhythmia that cannot be treated with painless therapy. (For more details on how ATP works, please see Chapter 2.)

VT ABLATION

Your doctor may also suggest that you undergo a procedure called an **ablation** to eliminate your VT. Because an arrhythmia is caused by electrical impulses traveling down an abnormal pathway, sometimes doctors can identify these pathways and "burn" them during an ablation procedure. (More information about ablation is available in Chapter 3.)

Chapter 9

Living with a Device

Throughout this book, you have learned a great deal about the physical and medical aspects of living with an ICD, pacemaker, or heart failure device. For those of you with an ICD or heart failure device that includes a defibrillator (CRT-D), understanding why you need the ICD, how it functions, and what to expect after implant will certainly help you and your family adjust and return to life more quickly. And the more experience you have living fully with the device, the more confident and peaceful you will likely become.

The good news is that multiple studies have shown that most ICD patients and families react very positively to the ICD; they report well-maintained, and often improved, quality of life after implant. But getting an ICD is not a minor event. Even the strongest of people may struggle with feelings of sadness, anxiety, and anger when their health changes or when they face a medical procedure. In fact, one out of every three ICD patients experience significant anxiety or depression at some point after ICD implant. They find it hard to feel secure and peaceful with having the ICD as a permanent fixture in their lives.

COPING MATTERS

Fortunately, for most ICD patients, as confidence in living with the device grows, negative feelings subside. This is important because positive emotions (like happiness, confidence, and hope) can help you to adjust positively to the device. In fact, research has shown that having an optimistic outlook on your health actually improves overall well-being and may improve your adjustment to the ICD. Also remember that your relationships matter, a bunch! Patients who receive emotional support from family and friends recover more quickly from all types of medical procedures and have better overall health outcomes.

ARE YOU AT RISK?

In addition to the general stress that comes with having a health concern, ICD patients face a variety of specific coping challenges post-implant that can lead to anxiety and/or depression. It is important to address these issues if they do occur, as mismanaged anxiety and depression can complicate your health. We will address ICD-specific coping challenges shortly, but let's first clarify what we mean by **anxiety** and **depression.**

Symptoms of Anxiety

Just about everyone knows what it's like to worry and feel anxious. But, for some, anxiety is a way of life, and chronic anxiety can complicate your health. For some of you or your loved ones with an ICD, we are referring to excessive worry that lasts for several months. The term "excessive" means that the level of worry is beyond what would be expected for a particular situation or event. If you are an "excessive worrier," you probably also have excessive anxiety, the kind of anxiety that makes it difficulty for you to relax and feel in control. Different people show different signs of problematic anxiety. In the list that follows, make a note of any symptom of anxiety that applies to you on a regular basis:

- Restlessness

- Fatigue

- Sleep disturbances

- Irritability

- Muscle tension

- Difficulty concentrating

- Nervousness

- Excessive fearfulness

- Obsessive worrying

Of course, everyone may experience some of these symptoms at one time or another. However, if anxiety symptoms are interfering with your daily functioning or causing you significant distress for a prolonged period of time, you may need special help.

Unfortunately, pride keeps many people from seeking help when it comes to anxiety or depression. It is important to keep in mind that you are only human. It is completely normal to have a period of adjustment after a major change in your life. Many of you have lived for decades without ever thinking twice about your health. Now, you are being confronted with not only your health, but perhaps thoughts of your own mortality as well.

All of us would be frightened to learn that we are at risk for sudden cardiac arrest. It is certainly normal to experience anxiety at the thought of having a cardiac arrhythmia. The physical symptoms of an arrhythmia (racing heart, rapid breathing, dizziness) may also induce feelings of anxiety. On top of that, you are living with a device that may deliver a high voltage shock without warning to terminate one of these life-threatening arrhythmias. Needless to say, it's natural and logical that some patients struggle to feel good about receiving an ICD.

The great news is that anxiety is very treatable and does not have to be a part of your daily life just because you have an ICD. Every day, thousands of people are helped to cope with anxiety through talk therapy, relaxation exercises, visual imagery exercises, anti-anxiety and anti-depressant medications, or any combination of these. Keep your physician informed about any anxiety symptoms that you or your family members may experience.

Speaking of family members, it's often the case that family members experience just as much, if not more, anxiety than the patient. Be patient with your family if this is the case, and remember that they may not understand exactly what you are feeling. You have the benefit of knowing how it feels to live through this difficult situation first-hand, while they don't. If you are a family member of a patient with a device and are experiencing anxiety, understand that this is a common occurrence. Seek help just as the patient would. It is often just as hard to deal with the mortality of those close to you as it is to grapple with your own mortality. (More information for family members and spouses of ICD patients can be found later in this chapter.)

Symptoms of Depression

Depression, if left untreated, is a significant health risk. Depression not only feels bad, it also compromises your body's ability to cope and to heal. There is strong evidence that depression may even complicate recovery from heart disease. Some symptoms of depression are fairly obvious and easy to identify, while others are more subtle. Know the symptoms of depression, and stay aware of any symptoms you may be experiencing.

Read through these obvious and subtle signs of depression and check any that apply to you:

- On most days, I feel hopeless and disinterested in activities that I typically find to be stimulating and enjoyable.

- I seem to have lost interest in activities that I normally find to be pleasurable.
- I have much less sex drive than usual.
- I feel indifferent and passive about facing my problems.
- In recent weeks, my appetite patterns have changed markedly, and my weight has changed significantly (gained or lost weight).
- My sleep patterns have changed in one or more of these ways: insomnia (difficulty falling asleep), disrupted sleep (difficulty staying asleep), or sleeping more hours than normal.
- I have much nervous energy.
- My muscles feel sluggish.
- I feel unusually fatigued, like I'm "stuck," and I have no energy to do anything about it.
- I feel inadequate and guilty.
- I am having difficulty thinking, concentrating, remembering, or making decisions.
- I am preoccupied with thoughts of death or suicide.

If you checked any five of these symptoms, and if you have been feeling this way more often than not for the past several weeks, you may be suffering from **clinical depression**. This is the sort of depression that can be dangerous to your health, and it requires medical attention.

Remember that depression, just like anxiety, is a very treatable condition, and like other health concerns, *it is not your fault*. Seek treatment just like you would any other health issue. You do not have to live with depressive symptoms, and you certainly do not have to face depression alone. Talk with your physician about any symptoms of depression you or your loved ones may experience. Good treatment options here include counseling, exercise, support groups, and anti-depressant medications.

We close this section with a word of encouragement. As already mentioned, anxiety and depression are treatable and, often, curable. If you have a history of anxiety, depression, or other mental health disturbances, you should let your physician know the specifics of your diagnosis and treatment. Particularly during the first months after your implant, or a change in your condition, you may need additional support and counseling to get you onto a positive coping path. Remember: Your emotions matter! You will adjust better to your ICD if you take good care of your psychological and emotional self. Doing so is every bit as important as taking care of your physical self.

This concept may be new to some of you. There once was a time that depression and anxiety, or any mental health issues for that matter, were viewed as signs of weakness. However, scientific knowledge is expanding, and we are learning that these psychological disturbances are a unique form of illness that affects many people worldwide. You should not feel ashamed, embarrassed, or guilty if you experience anxiety or depression in the wake of a heart disease diagnosis. This type of psychological struggle is not your fault and is not something you have to face alone.

POSSIBLE ADJUSTMENT DIFFICULTIES

Lifestyle Changes

The goal of ICD therapy is to enable you to live a full, long life, participating in all of the activities you enjoy. Although there are some activities that are not recommended with an ICD (see Chapter 5 for more information), most daily activities are safe. As mentioned in Chapter 5, some professions, such as a commercial airline pilot or commercial truck driver, are considered unsafe for ICD patients. If you are forced to change or terminate your profession as a result of getting an ICD, this will understandably present an adjustment challenge for you and your family. A job or profession often helps define a person, so losing this part of you may cause feelings of sadness, loss, and anger. These are all normal reactions to change. Consider talking with family and friends, or seek support from a mental health provider if possible. Remember that getting an ICD does not represent the end of your quality of life. It simply represents a new period in your life that may be challenging, but can also be rewarding and fulfilling.

Trusting Your Device

One of the most important steps toward living a full life with an ICD is learning to trust that your ICD is keeping you safe. For many patients, it takes time and effort to develop this trust. It is normal to at first struggle with the thought of having a machine implanted in your body. You may have doubts that the ICD will function properly. As discussed in Chapter 7, because ICDs are man-made devices, the possibility of a malfunction does exist. However, the overwhelming odds are that the ICD is going to function properly to successfully defibrillate your heart when necessary to save your life.

Many patients not only distrust their device, they actually blame their ICD for their health problems. This seems to be particularly prominent in patients who have an unexpected implant. One day you are normal and healthy (at least you thought you were), and the next day, you have this machine in your chest. It is important to remember that your ICD is not to blame for these extra worries and issues in your life. Your heart condition is. Your ICD helps to keep you alive, given that your heart disease puts you at risk for sudden cardiac arrest. As mentioned before, there are very few things that your ICD will prevent you from doing, but your heart condition may keep you from certain activities. Try to avoid "blaming" the ICD for any negative emotions or lifestyle adjustments you experience. Remember that your device may save your life someday.

Your thoughts about the ICD, whether positive or negative, can directly affect your feelings. Take notice of your thoughts about your device. Notice any negative thoughts and turn them into positive statements. Practice replacing negative statements such as, "I am scared that my ICD will not work properly," with positive statements such as "I know my ICD is keeping my heart safe." By learning about your ICD, you can understand how it functions to protect your heart and prolong your life. Remind yourself that the ICD is your best protection against cardiac arrest.

Body Image

Concern about body image after ICD implant is fairly common, especially among young patients and female patients. Because the ICD is usually implanted just under the skin in the chest area, the outline of the device may be visible. Some patients say they feel uncomfortable wearing certain shirts or bathing suits that reveal the slight bulge beneath their skin, where their device is implanted. Others let self-consciousness about the device hinder their social life or leisure activities (such as going to the beach or pool).

If you are like the vast majority of people, although it may take some time, you *will* become comfortable with the ICD and accept it as a special form of protection housed in your body. In fact, many patients become so comfortable that they no longer notice the device or even think about its presence. As with most life changes, learning to feel comfortable with the ICD may simply take time and a little effort on your part.

Another adjustment may be dealing with the questions from others about your device. Many patients report that they don't feel comfortable at a public swimming pool, not because they aren't "sexy" anymore, but rather because they don't like to answer the question, "What's that?" regarding the bulge where their device sits. Whether the question is asked by an inquisitive child or adolescent, or by a less sensitive adult, it's probably best to simply respond that it's a small machine that helps to support your heart. The question likely isn't meant to invade your privacy, so try not to be bothered when these questions arise.

Living with a Device

Take heart (and coping lessons) from one of our patients.

Karen was a 42-year-old woman who felt very self-conscious about the visibility of her ICD. She would even avoid letting her husband see her body due to her insecurities. Every time she looked in the mirror, Karen focused on the bulge of her ICD and became upset. But one day, a passing comment by a friend helped her to put this into perspective:

"I was complaining to my friend Susan, and she said something interesting: 'Karen, you've been self-conscious about one part or another of your body for the entire time I've known you. I so wish for you that you'd let yourself come to peace with yourself.'

"Susan's comment hit me like a ton of bricks! I realized how true it was that, for most of my life, I criticized how I looked. Focusing on this little bulge was just the latest version of my habit.

"My second 'aha' came one day while I was listening to a radio talk show while driving my kids to school. The person being interviewed kept saying 'Happiness is a choice.' My 14-year-old son started making fun of the phrase, and the more silly he got, the more I realized how much sense this actually made. Happiness *is* a choice, and I had been choosing to deny it. For most of my life, the culprit that ruined my happiness was my focusing on how my body was not perfect. That radio show helped me to realize that, all along, my own criticism and lack of acceptance of myself was the real problem, not my body.

"I'm not saying that I changed all of this. I do still struggle some with my insecurities. But I have been practicing—and that's the right word, literally: practicing—being kinder to myself. I remind myself each day that the little bulge beneath my skin is a 'guardian angel' looking after my heart health. I remind myself what I can do and try to focus less on what I might avoid doing, just because I don't have a perfect body. I have my ups and downs. But I have more good days now than ever before."

Do your best to notice any negative thoughts you have about how the ICD looks or feels in your body, and remind yourself that it is there to help you live a longer, safer life. If you are having extreme difficulty accepting your ICD, talk to your doctor or someone else you trust about these feelings. You may benefit from talking with a mental health provider who specializes in body image concerns.

YOUNG PATIENTS

"Young" ICD patients are usually defined as 50 years old and younger, although there have also been infants who have required ICDs. Those of you who are younger may have a more difficult time adjusting to life with an ICD for several reasons. First, receiving an ICD may serve as a reminder of your mortality. This sort of wake-up call is difficult enough for older patients, but it seems untimely for someone who is young. Young people may have a sense of entitlement about good health—that is, they assume they will stay healthy for a long time, and they may even take this for granted. Learning that you need an ICD can rattle this sense of security in your own good health. Furthermore, young ICD patients may feel especially alone in their struggle. Since most ICD patients are in their 60s or older, younger patients sometimes say they have trouble finding peers with whom they can connect. If this is the case, ask your healthcare provider if they can help you find a "young" ICD support group. There are several weekend-long support groups designed for young people with devices. Seek one out. Or simply get online! (See Appendix 1 for suggested websites.)

Young ICD patients may also have a difficult time accepting any lifestyle restrictions that come along with heart disease or ICD implant. Young patients are often still active individuals who are working and raising families. They may have fears about what their children will think about the ICD, and whether the possibility of witnessing a shock will scare them. Young ICD patients also report more concerns about passing their heart condition to their children.

If you are a younger patient and any of these concerns sound familiar to you, first know that your feelings are likely a normal part of the adjustment process after ICD implant. As stated earlier, it will take some work on your part, but you *can* develop positive feelings about your ICD. Instead of focusing on how the ICD has had a negative impact on your life, try to recognize the positive facts: In previous times, you would likely have died from a heart condition that can now be treated with ICD therapy. Fortunately, medicine has advanced enough to allow earlier diagnosis of potentially fatal heart conditions. Although it may feel untimely and unnatural to have an ICD at a young age, this technology will likely allow you to live a longer, safer, fuller life than you would have without the ICD. Remember to acknowledge your feelings about the ICD, keep your healthcare providers informed about how you are adjusting, and seek guidance from a mental health provider if necessary. If you have the opportunity to connect with another young ICD patient, do so. Often just talking with a peer, or someone who is going through a similar challenge, can energize you and give you a fresh perspective. Your insights will also be valuable to other ICD patients.

COPING WITH SHOCKS

You have read a good deal about shock throughout this book. By now, we trust that you understand how a shock might save your life by stopping an arrhythmia and putting your heart back into a normal rhythm. But being shocked is not just a physical event; there also may be psychological impacts of a shock experience. No one likes to be shocked. In fact, most patients say they worry about being shocked. Whether or not they have ever actually received a shock, they struggle with the fear of pain from a shock, loss of control, and embarrassment they may feel if they receive a shock in public.

Research has shown that ICD patients who receive one or more shocks report lower quality of life and more depression and anxiety than do patients who haven't received a shock. Some studies show that regardless of age, sex, or the other risk factors we have mentioned, shock alone predicts which patients will experience emotional struggles. And some patients who have experienced one shock or multiple shocks suffer from anxiety or panic symptoms when they remember the experience. Let's elaborate on this last scenario.

Patients with multiple shock experiences are more likely to develop an anxiety condition called **post-traumatic stress disorder (PTSD)**. PTSD refers to a collection of symptoms that may occur after a traumatic experience. These symptoms include, but are not limited to:

- Intrusive Thoughts—repeated thoughts of the frightening event; may interfere with concentration or daily functioning
- Avoidance Behaviors—avoiding particular places, situations, people, or emotions because you associate them with the shock experience
- Hyperarousal—physical symptoms of extreme anxiety: irritability, nightmares, panic attacks, strong startle response

The symptoms of PTSD can be very distressing and can interfere with your ability to function. If you experience any of these symptoms at any time, alert your nurse or physician. PTSD is a very treatable condition, but usually requires several sessions of therapy with a mental health provider.

Jan was a 55-year-old woman who received an ICD a year after having a heart attack. After implant, Jan reported feeling well and was able to quickly return to her daily routines. One important part of Jan's life was her weekly trips to Walmart. She enjoyed the trips and the fact that the store was convenient to her home and carried most of the household items she needed. A few months after ICD implant, Jan received three shocks while shopping in her local Walmart. She was understandably shaken by this episode, but was comforted to hear that the shocks were likely preventable in the future by adjusting some of her ICD settings. Jan reported feeling a little embarrassed about the shock episode happening in such a public place. She also indicated that, while the shocks were happening, she felt fearful about dying. Despite her fears, Jan still felt confident that the ICD would save her life if necessary, and she recovered well. However, she refused to revisit her local Walmart. Jan understood that the shocks did not happen because of her environment— in other words, there was nothing about Walmart that triggered her device to shock. However, Jan associated the store with her frightening, traumatic experience, and was therefore unwilling to return. She chose instead to drive 15 miles to the next town's Walmart. As Jan explained one day, "I don't feel like I have any control over this device. I don't control if or when it shocks me. But I can control which Walmart I go to, and I am no longer comfortable in my local store." Jan's behavior represents a classic avoidance scenario. She used to enjoy her local Walmart, but now fears and avoids it because she associates it with being shocked.

PLANNING FOR A SHOCK

The most difficult part of living with an ICD may be the fact that you are not in control of what your device does. Many patients report that it is hard to accept the fact that the device may deliver a shock at any time, without warning, and that they have no control over when that will happen.

It is exhausting and unproductive to focus your energy on situations that are out of your control. This can only lead to further frustration. A good alternative is to focus your energy on factors you can control, including how to prepare yourself and your family for a potential shock situation. Developing a "shock plan" can benefit you and your family members by clarifying the steps you will take if an ICD shock occurs in a variety of scenarios. The basic steps of shock planning are described below.

Step One: Talk to Your Doctor

The first step in making a shock plan is to talk to your physician about what he or she recommends you do if you receive an ICD shock. The recommendations may differ, depending on whether you have symptoms at the time of shock (such as shortness of breath, dizziness, chest pain), and whether you have received one shock or more than one shock. Typically, if you have received more than one shock within 24 hours, this is considered an emergency situation for which you should seek immediate medical attention. Your physician will also want to interrogate your ICD after a shock, but some situations may not require immediate attention. Be sure you know and understand your physician's recommendations around this issue.

Step Two: Talk to Family and Friends

The next step in planning for shock is to talk to your family or friends about how they can help you respond if you receive a shock. It may be helpful to identify a few family members or neighbors you could call at any hour to drive you to the hospital if necessary, or to take care of things at home while you seek medical care. Write down names and phone numbers of these people and keep them in your wallet with your device ID card, or some other convenient location, along with instructions from your physician. You may also want to display their contact information, as well as contact information for your physician's office and hospital, on your refrigerator or somewhere else visible in your house. Identifying these people to help you in an emergent situation may further reduce your anxiety around shock.

You should also talk to these friends and family members about their responses if you should lose consciousness. For the most part, patients with ICDs usually regain consciousness within seconds, but still it's good to remind family and friends that it's okay to touch you during a shock. A sensation could be felt by someone touching an ICD patient during a shock. However, it wouldn't be dangerous in any way and while it might feel unusual, it likely would not be painful. Also, remind them that if you do lose consciousness, while the device will likely react and you will regain consciousness, they need to be prepared to seek help—that is, call 911—if needed. It's important to take immediate steps to get medical help for anyone who has lost consciousness, whether they have an ICD or not. On the flip side, a call to 911 is definitely not needed for every shock if you recover without incident. If you feel well, proceed as described in this chapter.

Furthermore, discuss and plan for what your family should do in an emergency. Consider every aspect of the situation: What hospital do you want to go to? Do you want your family to ride along in the ambulance, or stay home and take care of the dog? Where is your current list of medications, or a quick medical summary if paramedics or caregivers need it? Having these seemingly minor issues resolved will go a long way toward keeping your calm during an episode, should you ever have one.

Step Three: Plan Your Own Response

A final, and very important, step in shock planning is thinking about how you will respond to a shock in ways that will calm you and keep you focused. Depending on where you are when you receive an ICD shock, it may be helpful to lie down and breathe deeply. Regardless of what you are doing when you received the shock, slowing down and taking deep breaths will start to calm both your mind and your body. Relaxing your muscles will also reduce any lingering feelings of pain from the shock. You should also make an effort to think positive thoughts during this time. Remind yourself that the ICD is there to protect you. Shocks may happen, but they are not necessarily a sign of trouble. Tell yourself that, although shock may be scary and uncomfortable, the ICD is your best protection against sudden cardiac death. Perhaps one thing that may be helpful to ask yourself, even during an event, is simply, "Would I rather my ICD *wasn't* going off?" Even though lying in the middle of a sidewalk or a store getting a shock may seem like the worst thing possible, it's not as bad as the alternative, which would likely be death.

An important part of maintaining your quality of life after a shock involves planning for how you will return to doing all the things you enjoy, even if the shock experience has caused you to fear certain activities. It is logical to assume that you may be anxious about engaging in activities that remind you of being shocked. However, unless your physician or device nurse has instructed you not to participate in an activity, you *can* and *should* return to doing what you enjoy. Otherwise, you are at risk for developing negative emotions if you stop living your life to the fullest. It bears repeating: Unless your physician or device nurse has instructed you not to participate in an activity, you *can* and *should* return to doing what you enjoy. Don't let your ICD keep you alive, yet steal your life.

SPOUSES OF ICD PATIENTS

Throughout this chapter, you have learned about the importance of watching for signs of psychological distress in yourself as well as in your family members. Family members of ICD patients, especially spouses, play an important role in the recovery process after ICD implant. Research indicates that caregivers can improve outcomes of cardiovascular patients, particularly when they support the patient in making healthy lifestyle changes and coping with the emotional effects of heart disease.

However, being the spouse or caregiver of an ICD patient can also be a stressful, perhaps frightening, experience. In fact, studies indicate that spouses of ICD patients experience as much anxiety and concern about ICD implant as patients do, and often even more. In our experience, ICD patients sometimes have an easier time accepting the ICD and mentally recover from the experience more quickly than their spouses do.

Simply put, the caregiver role can be exhausting and overwhelming. Your spouse and family members may be bothered by the memory of events surrounding the device implant, particularly if they witnessed you having a cardiac arrest episode or a heart attack. Remember, while you were uncon-scious, they were watching someone they love dearly walk the line between life and death.

Your spouse or family members may also be more concerned about the recovery process than you are. They may have more anxiety about your making lifestyle changes, regulating medications, traveling, or returning to work. Also, many families are uncomfortable leaving the patient alone after implant.

> After her husband Joe received an ICD, Mary found that she was suddenly afraid to leave him alone for long periods of time. Mary was concerned about what would happen if Joe received an ICD shock and she wasn't there to take care of him. Before Joe got the ICD, Mary was very social, and an avid bridge player. After Joe's implant, however, Mary rarely saw her friends and had not yet resumed attending bridge games. She missed her "fun" time, but felt obligated to stay home with Joe just in case something should happen.
>
> Subsequently, Mary's quality of life began to suffer. She felt extremely anx-ious. In fact, it seemed that she was more anxious and concerned about living with an ICD than Joe was. Although it was difficult for her to admit, Mary also felt somewhat angry and resentful that she seemed to be bearing the emotional burden of this process even though Joe was the one with an ICD!

This scenario occurs commonly, particularly among spouses of ICD pa-tients. Caregiver strain is a very real phenomenon that can have negative emotional and physical effects. As a spouse or caregiver to an ICD patient, you may be concerned about a number of things that we have addressed in this chapter. It is essential that you acknowledge your own needs and feelings as you and your family adjust to life with an ICD. Stay aware of the symptoms of anxiety and depression in yourself. Take time to engage in activities you enjoy that are outside your "caregiver" role. Spend time alone, participate in your hobbies, and socialize with your friends. Take comfort in the fact that your family member is protected by the ICD at all times. In fact, he or she is safer now than before the ICD implant! You may also benefit from talking with spouses of other patients (for example, in an ICD support group). You may learn a great deal simply by hearing how other families have coped with this adjustment process.

Chapter 10

Other Important Issues

This chapter provides information on two topics that may cause confusion and a mix of emotions for any device patient. These topics are device advisories and decisions that need to be made regarding an implantable device when you or your family member with a device is facing a terminal illness or end-of-life decisions.

DEVICE ADVISORIES

In order to live a full, thriving life with an ICD, you must learn to accept and trust that the device is protecting you. As mentioned in Chapter 9, some patients have a hard time putting trust in a man-made device. Patients may struggle with having to rely on a piece of machinery for their physical well-being. This may be especially true if you are concerned about the possibility of a specific warning or alert (most appropriately called an "advisory") being issued for your device or one of your leads. You have likely heard about advisories, sometimes called "recalls," of heart devices or leads in the news at some point. This is a topic that gets a significant amount of media coverage when it occurs. Unfortunately, the amount of media coverage is often disproportionate to the number of people who are actually affected by these advisories. An advisory or recall may also be brought to your attention by legal firms advertising for patients who have such a device or lead, in the hope of convincing them to be part of a class-action lawsuit.

The number of medical device advisories has increased significantly in recent years. However, this is not because devices are less well made than they used to be. On the contrary, the number of advisories has increased in part because devices are increasingly complex and advanced. However, when devices have more features and intricacies, there are more features that can potentially have problems.

Advisories also occur at times for pacemaker or ICD leads. This may be related to a problem with the durability of the lead, which could be related to the initial design. Despite rigorous testing of the leads prior to being approved for use, some problems simply don't become apparent until a lead has been in the body and functioning for long periods of time.

Another reason for the increase in medical device advisories is that the device companies are held to a much stricter standard than ever before when it comes to requirements to report any issues or problems with their products. Companies are required to issue an advisory if even an extremely small percentage of devices or leads are affected by it. An advisory may be issued for problems that are not immediately life-threatening. Regardless of the reason for the advisory, if your device or lead is affected, you may initially experience fear and concern.

Research on how patients react to advisory announcements is limited, and the results are mixed. Most studies show that when an advisory is announced, it is common for patients to experience concern and some level of fear, even if they learn that their device or leads are not affected. The situation may make you feel vulnerable because it highlights the fact that devices and leads are not perfect. Your family members may also be affected by an advisory. They may experience anxiety and decreased confidence in your device or leads. However, for the majority of patients and their family members, these feelings are temporary. We know that most patients do quite well after an advisory announcement, even if they are directly affected by it.

Research indicates that your reaction to an advisory may depend on how you first receive the news. Most patients would like to hear about an advisory during a conversation with their doctor or nurse. However, the vast majority of patients first hear about an advisory through the media. This is a difficult situation to change or control, because as soon as an advisory is known to or issued by the government, it becomes public information that the media can distribute. Often, the doctors will learn about the advisory from the device companies, but it is difficult for the doctor or the clinic to get the news to all their patients before patients hear it elsewhere. Many patients end up hearing about an advisory on the news or from other patients. This can increase fear and anxiety because you may not get all of the information, or the accurate information, about exactly what types of devices or leads are affected. Therefore, regardless of the specifics, you may all feel vulnerable and scared by this news.

It is important to remember that the chance of your device or leads having a serious malfunction or defect is extremely small. There is a much greater chance that your device will function normally and will enable you to live a longer, safer life. Of course it is true that everything man-made is susceptible to defects. Just like your car, your computer, and your washing machine, your device is a machine with many parts. Sometimes machine parts need to be changed or fixed, and this may be true for your device or leads as well. Naturally, experiencing a problem with your heart device is a much more personal, emotional issue than dealing with a broken washing machine. But accepting that devices and leads are imperfect is an important part of having a realistic outlook on this process.

Recently there has been a great deal of media coverage about alerts and advisories on pacemakers and/or ICDs and/or specific leads. As a result of this attention, patients who were told they needed a device, either new or replacement, were appropriately concerned and would ask many questions about the risk of a problem for whatever system they were going to have implanted. If you have questions about the safety of the products you will receive, remember that if a product already has an advisory or alert issued, then almost certainly that product has been removed from the hospitals and is no longer being implanted. It is important and appropriate for you and your loved ones to be proactive in asking questions about these issues. However, sometimes patients have insisted on having a device that is guaranteed to never have an advisory or other problem, or the patient only wants products coming from a company that has never issued an advisory. It's important to understand that all device manufacturers have, at some point, had an advisory or other alert about a problem affecting one or more of their products. In order to choose a product that will never fail, the doctor would need a crystal ball to predict the future, and obviously that's not possible. Caregivers and patients do have access to reports from the device manufacturers that describe how well a specific product has performed to date, but that's really the best information out there. As noted above, no man-made product or machine is perfect. For that matter, your own equipment—that is, your heart—isn't always guaranteed to function perfectly either. If it were, there would be no reason to discuss the need for a device to be implanted!

If you are affected by an advisory or recall, trust that your doctors, nurses, and the device company are going to respond in the most appropriate way for your individual situation. It is difficult, but if you hear about an advisory on the news, try not to get too worried. Depending on what type of advisory it is, your doctor may decide that no action is necessary, or perhaps the issue can be fixed or minimized with the programmer in the doctor's office.

As mentioned earlier, many advisories are relatively minor issues that do not require devices or leads to be removed. It may be that your doctor will simply need to re-program some settings on your device or have your device and leads monitored more frequently. In some cases, device or lead removal or replacement may be recommended for certain patients, depending on their type of heart disease. However, there are always risks associated with undergoing another surgery. It is ultimately up to the doctor to discuss this with you. Together you can decide what the best treatment option is for your individual situation. What is best for you may not be what is best for another patient with the same device.

The fact that advisory situations do occur reinforces the importance of having your device followed regularly. When your device is checked, whether in the doctor's office or using your remote monitor, your healthcare provider is able to see some very important information about how the device is functioning. If there is a problem with your device or leads, your healthcare provider may be able to see this during a routine follow-up. Missing follow-up appointments or failing to send your scheduled remote transmissions increases the chances that a problem with your device or leads will go undetected. The best way to stay safe and confident that your device is working properly is to receive regular follow-up. Hopefully this will give you the peace of mind to return to your life feeling secure and protected by your heart device.

END-OF-LIFE DECISIONS

If you are like most patients, at some point since you were told that you need a heart device, you have had thoughts about your own mortality. When faced with a new diagnosis, illness, or surgery, people tend to think about how and when their lives will end. This is a difficult topic for many people to discuss and may even be disturbing for you to think about. It may seem strange to talk about or think about death when you are trying to feel thankful for the life-saving therapy you are receiving from your heart device. However, end-of-life issues are concerning for many patients and, unfortunately, often go unaddressed for far too long. In fact, research indicates that many doctors do not bring up discussions about end-of-life treatment with patients until the patient is already nearing death. Research on patients' and family members' preferences indicates that many would rather discuss this topic ahead of time, long before they are faced with having to make decisions about end-of-life management.

You may have questions about how your heart device will function when you are dying. Many patients wonder if the device will keep them alive forever, or at least keep their heart beating even if they are technically "dead." It is a good idea to ask your doctor all of these questions anytime you are discussing device therapy. The best way for you and your family to be prepared for this emotional situation is to understand all your options.

Can I Request My Device Be Turned Off?

The law in the United States clearly states that if a patient, or the person designated to make medical decisions on behalf of the patient, wants a device turned "off," it is indeed the patient's right to have to this done. The caregivers involved would want to carefully document your request in the medical record, talk to you or your medical decision maker about other options that may be considered, and explain how turning off a device or specific portions of the therapies will or will not have an immediate effect on you. Not all caregivers are comfortable turning off a device. Caregivers cannot be forced to do something with which they are not comfortable. However, it is their responsibility to find someone else who would adhere to your wishes and to do so in a timely manner.

If you have a pacemaker, you may understand that the pacemaker can deliver electrical impulses to keep your heart beating. This process works very well in a living, viable heart muscle. However, if no changes are made to your pacemaker and if you die from other causes, your heart tissue is therefore "dead," meaning it will no longer respond to electrical impulses from the pacemaker. The pacemaker will not keep a deceased patient alive. Often, but not always, after a person dies, a doctor, nurse, technician, or a representative from the device company will turn the pacemaker off so that it no longer delivers impulses.

The pacemaker can also be turned off when it is determined that you are dying and you no longer wish to receive life-sustaining treatment. If the pacemaker is turned off, that simply means it will not deliver electrical impulses to the heart, even if the heart stops beating. Turning off a pacemaker does not necessarily mean that you are going to die within minutes. If you are not dependent on the pacemaker to keep your heart beating, meaning that your own heartbeat comes through when the pacemaker isn't functioning, turning off the pacemaker would not have any immediate effect. If you are dependent on the pacemaker, turning it off would likely result in an immediate death.

End-of-life care for ICD patients is a little more complex. The basic principles still apply: If you are dead and no longer have functioning heart tissue, the ICD will not keep you alive. For ICD patients, the main concern about dying is the thought of being shocked multiple times as they are dying and their heart is failing. This scenario is possible if the ICD is left on during death. As with pacemaker patients, if it is determined that you are close to death and you wish to remove some life-saving measures, you may have your ICD turned off. "Turning off" an ICD is essentially forcing the device to close its eyes. The ICD will not recognize or treat any life-threatening arrhythmias once it has been programmed off. Therefore, if you experienced ventricular fibrillation, which is a life-threatening arrhythmia, the ICD would not intervene to treat it, and you would likely die within a few minutes. For many patients, this is a much more peaceful death scenario than having the device shock them in an attempt to stop the fast heart rhythm. Again, as with pacemaker patients, it is unlikely that you would die immediately after the ICD is turned off. Programming the device off does nothing to increase the chances that you will experience an arrhythmia. It just means that the device will not treat an arrhythmia if one occurs. Since all ICDs include a pacemaker, turning off the portion of the ICD that treats the fast heart rhythms does not necessarily mean turning off the pacemaker. If you or a loved one is facing such a decision, talk with your caregivers about the options available.

Cardiac resynchronization therapy devices can also be turned off, if that is the option you or your medical decision maker desire. Turning off the resynchronization portion of the device may result in a worsening of your heart failure, but would likely not lead to any immediate dramatic change in status.

It is important that you understand that device deactivation is *not* the same as physician-assisted suicide. Turning off a device will not be the cause of death for any patient. It simply means that life-saving treatment will be withheld if the patient begins to die. The heart problem that led the patient to get a device is what really causes death, not the machine's inability to restore a rhythm after it's turned off. Turning off a device is not all that different from enacting a **do not resuscitate order** restricting healthcare workers from using a defibrillator or CPR to revive you.

Once a patient with an ICD is deceased, the ICD can be turned off to avoid delivery of any therapy or emission of any alert tones. However, this isn't an absolute requirement. Additionally, if the patient is going to be cremated, it will be necessary to remove the ICD, pacemaker, or cardiac resynchronization device before this is done.

Planning End-of-Life Care

The acronym **NEEDS** may help you remember the important steps in making your plans for end-of-life care. This acronym was developed to encourage patients to think about and discuss these issues with their loved ones:[1]

Notify your loved ones of your wishes for end-of-life care related to your device, and document them legally.

Educate yourself about treatment options.

Evaluate all of your treatment options.

Discuss your preferences and consider palliative care.

Seek mental and spiritual health care to aid in this difficult time.

In terms of legally documenting your wishes, this does not have to be complicated or expensive and does not require legal representation. Your caregiver likely has access to a document that will allow you to formalize your wishes in your medical records. This is often referred to as an **advance directive.** If your caregiver does not have an advance directive document available, they should be able to direct you to other sources. There are some excellent web sites and print material available about advance directives that you or your family members should be able to access relatively easily. (The "do not resuscitate" order, or DNR, mentioned earlier is one type of advance directive.)

Make these decisions and talk to your family members while you are still able to do so. In the absence of documenting your wishes, it will make things even more difficult for family members or loved ones facing a difficult time. It goes back to the NEEDS acronym described above. If someone is dying from a terminal illness, such as the final days of heart failure or a cancer that can no longer be treated, ongoing pain and suffering may outweigh any benefits of continuing therapy offered from an implantable device.

[1] Sears et al., PACE, 2006; 29: 637–642.

Another situation that can be very difficult for family members occurs when the person with the device has developed severe dementia or Alzheimer's disease. A common scenario is that the patient who has developed severe dementia has a device that reaches battery depletion and needs replacement. Such individuals are faced with extremely poor quality of life; they often reside in a care facility and may no longer be able to recognize friends and family. Family members may be reluctant to even ask whether it would be appropriate to consider *not* replacing the device. In this situation, if the patient's documented wishes include what to do in the event of dementia, the family or loved ones know how to proceed. In the absence of an advance directive that is specific to the situation, it is common to hear family members make comments like, "We know (Mom or Dad) would not want to live like this, but would we feel right if we decide not to have the device replaced?" For such a patient, often elderly, the situation is sometimes made even worse when children turn to the spouse of the patient—the person who may be having the most difficult time with the decision—and ask, "Do you know what he/she would want us to do?" As previously noted, these are tough and emotional conversations to have, but it's important to have them ahead of time in the event such a situation arises.

When it comes to expressing your wishes, to whatever degree you are comfortable doing so, you should be as specific as possible. Sometimes it's difficult for family members or loved ones to interpret statements such as "Do nothing heroic . . ." because ideas about what "heroic" means differ. Specific to your implantable device, after seeking advice from some or all of the individuals above, consider the statements below, which would be helpful to others who are trying to interpret your wishes.

In the event that I am unable to make my own decisions and am felt to have no meaningful chance of recovering, in regard to my (pacemaker/ICD/CRT) I want:

- Device left as is—OR
- Any "shocks" turned off—OR
- All treatments for fast heart rhythms, that is shocks or rapid pacing treatments, turned off—OR
- My device turned off completely, which includes all therapies for slow heart rates (my pacemaker), fast heart rates (my defibrillator), and heart failure (my CRT device).

Again, the more specific you can be and still feel comfortable with your decisions, the easier and clearer you will make it for those who are being asked to interpret your wishes.

All of this technical language may seem a little daunting when discussing such a sensitive topic. However, you and your family will hopefully experience peace of mind when you understand and discuss all your options. Many patients find that it is easier to have these conversations now, rather than waiting until a loved one is dying—a time when you are forced to make hard decisions in a stressful environment. Just as you may put other affairs in order—your power of attorney, your will, and so on—it makes sense to decide if and when you will have your device turned off as you near the end of your life. It may help to talk to a counselor, religious leader, or someone else you trust as you are working through these decisions.

Appendix I

Patient Resources Online

Patient Education Websites

American Heart Association
http://www.heart.org/HEARTORG/

Heart Rhythm Society
http://www.hrsonline.org/PatientInfo/

Device Manufacturer Websites

Biotronik
http://www.biotronik.com/wps/wcm/connect/en_us_web/biotronik/sub_
    top/patients/
503-635-3594

Boston Scientific
http://www.bostonscientific.com/home.bsci
800-227-3422

Medtronic
http://www.medtronic.com/health-consumers/index.htm
800-328-2518

St. Jude Medical
http://health.sjm.com/
800-328-9634

Sorin
http://www.sorin.com/anatomy
877-663-7674

Appendix 2

Understanding Abbreviations for Devices

You and your family will likely hear your healthcare providers talk in abbreviations as they talk about the type of device and/or how the device is programmed. These abbreviations may sound like somewhat of an alphabet soup the first time you hear them. The following terms should help you understand some fairly straightforward abbreviations that may otherwise seem mysterious.

DEVICE ABBREVIATIONS

PM—pacemaker

ICD—implantable cardioverter defibrillator

CRT—cardiac resynchronization therapy

CRT-P—CRT device with only pacing therapy

CRT-D—CRT device with an ICD incorporated

PACING MODE DESIGNATIONS

A code is used to describe different types of pacemakers or, more accurately, how an individual pacemaker is currently programmed. This code has been used for many years and consists of four letters. For example, the pacemaker in your device may be programmed "DDDR."

What Do the Letters Mean?

The first letter is for the chamber paced. If only the ventricle is paced, the first letter will be V. If only the atrium is paced, the first letter is A. If both chambers are paced, the first letter is D.

The second letter indicates how the pacemaker responds to the heart's native rhythm. It's usually important that the pacemaker be able to detect your natural heartbeat so that it only works when needed. Again, if the pacemaker senses ventricular activity, the letter V is used; if atrial activity is sensed, the letter A is used. If the pacemaker is sensing or "watching" your cardiac activity from both chambers, using a dual-chamber system, a D is used.

The third letter describes how the device responds when the patient's own heart activity is sensed. When your own heart activity is sensed and the pacemaker temporarily stops pacing, the letter I is used. If the patient's natural heartbeat results in the pacemaker putting out an impulse, the letter T is used. (This setting is almost never used in a single-chamber pacemaker.) If you have a dual-chamber device, the letter D may sometimes appear. This letter is used when activity in both your heart's atrium and ventricle inhibits the pacemaker (shown as an I, meaning **inhibited**) and your intrinsic atrial activity also stimulates the lower chamber.

The fourth letter indicates whether the pacemaker can alter the pacing rate based on your activity. If the device is capable of this, the letter R appears in the fourth position, indicating that the pacemaker is **rate responsive.** In other words, it is capable of adjusting your heart *rate* in *response* to your activity. If the pacemaker is not programmed to be rate responsive, the fourth position is left blank. Most devices do have this "rate-responsiveness" or "rate-adaptation" capability that can be turned on as needed. When this setting is turned on, the pacemaker will change the rate at which it paces your heart based on your activity, movement, and/or breathing rate and depth of breaths taken. For example, if you are sitting quietly or sleeping, and breathing normally, the pacemaker will only pace at the lowest rate setting. If you then start to move around and start breathing faster and deeper, the pacemaker will detect your activity and increase the pacing rate appropriately.

Some Examples

- A pacemaker that can pace and sense the upper chamber (atrium) only, is inhibited by your heart's atrial activity, and does not respond to changes in activity of some type = AAI
- A pacemaker that can pace and sense the lower chamber (ventricle) only, is inhibited by your own atrial activity, and does respond to changes in activity of some type = VVIR
- A pacemaker that can pace and sense in both the upper and lower chambers, is inhibited by your own activity in both chambers, can pace or stimulate the lower chamber whenever it senses activity in your upper chamber, and does respond to changes in activity of some type = DDDR

A FINAL NOTE

Many clinicians often will use these codes as a type of shorthand as well. Instead of saying "dual-chamber pacemaker," they may simply say "DDD pacer." Or they may call a single-chamber pacemaker a "VVI device."

Glossary

A

Antiarrhythmics—medicines designed to prevent or decrease cardiac arrhythmias.

Antitachycardia pacing (ATP)—very fast pacing delivered by an implanted heart device to treat an abnormally fast heartbeat.

Atrial fibrillation (AF)—a heart rhythm that causes the atria to quiver—that is, to lose all organized activity—rather than contract.

Atrial flutter—an atrial heart rhythm that is regular but very fast.

Atrial tachyarrhythmias—abnormally fast heart rhythms that start in the atria or upper chambers of the heart. Atrial flutter and atrial fibrillation are atrial tachyarrhythmias.

Atrioventricular node (AV node)—an area of cardiac muscle fibers located in the middle portion of the heart. Electrical signals from a different set of fibers located higher in the heart, the sinoatrial (SA) node, travel through the AV node before moving to the rest of the heart—that is, the lower chambers of the heart—or ventricles. The AV node helps keep the upper and lower heart chambers beating in a synchronized rhythm.

Atrium (plural = atria)—the two upper chambers of the heart are referred to as the right atrium and the left atrium. The term "atria" is the plural of "atrium" and refers to both the right and the left atrium.

Avoidance behaviors—avoiding particular places, situations, people, or emotions because of an association with a traumatic event.

B

Bipolar lead—a type of lead used with an implantable heart device that consists of two wires that are insulated from each other and insulated from the outside.

Biventricular (Bi-V) devices—See **Cardiac resynchronization therapy devices.**

Bradycardia—a type of heart condition in which the heart beats less than 60 beats per minute.

Bypass surgery—surgery to correct blocked coronary arteries—that is, the source of blood for the heart muscle. The complete name is "coronary artery bypass grafting," which is abbreviated CABG and which medical professionals refer to as "cabbage." The bypass may be made from veins taken from the legs, or sometimes an internal artery is disconnected from its original position and reattached to the coronary artery to supply blood flow.

C

Cardiac ablation—a procedure in which a very small portion of tissue in the heart is destroyed in an effort to control or cure an abnormal heart rhythm; performed by an electrophysiologist.

Cardiac resynchronization therapy devices (CRT devices)—used for patients with congestive heart failure and associated symptoms; a CRT device typically consists of three leads: one in each ventricle and one in the right atrium. CRT devices may be pacemakers (CRT-P) or ICDs (CRT-D). See also **Biventricular (Bi-V) devices.**

Cardioversion—a therapy to treat an extremely fast but stable heart rhythm. Cardioversion therapy involves delivering a low-level shock to the heart synchronized or in time with

your natural heartbeat. This therapy may increase to higher energy levels if the initial treatment is not successful. Cardioversion may be delivered by an implanted heart device (ICD), or in some patients without a device, an external cardioversion is performed.

Circumflex artery—one of three main coronary arteries. The circumflex artery circles around to the outside lateral wall of the left ventricle.

D

Defibrillation—a type of therapy provided by an implanted heart device or external electronic equipment to treat a fast, irregular heart rhythm. Defibrillation therapy involves delivering a high-energy therapy shock to the heart. As opposed to cardioversion, which is generally done for non-life-threatening heart rhythms, defibrillation is not "synchronized" to the native heart rhythm because the native heart rhythm is usually chaotic or extremely fast.

Defibrillation threshold testing (DFT)—a test performed during an ICD implant to define the amount of energy required for the ICD to successfully defibrillate the heart.

Defibrillator—an external or implanted device used to deliver defibrillation therapy to the heart.

Dual-chamber pacemaker—a pacemaker that uses two leads, usually placed in the right atrium and right ventricle (also called a DDD or DDDR pacemaker).

Glossary

E

ECG or EKG—ECG (EKG) is an abbreviation for "electrocardiogram." An electrocardiogram is a test that measures the electrical activity of a person's heart.

Echocardiogram—an ultrasound of the heart that assesses the pumping efficiency of the left ventricle, or LVEF (see also **Left ventricular ejection fraction**), as well as the heart valves and other structures of the heart.

Ejection fraction (EF)—the percentage or fraction of blood that the left ventricle squeezes out with each beat (see also **Left ventricular ejection fraction**) A normal EF is 50 to 60%.

Elective replacement indicator (ERI)—an indication of the remaining battery life of an implanted heart device; at ERI, a device has approximately 3 months of full battery usage available.

Electrocautery—a technique used during surgery to control bleeding.

Electromagnetic interference (EMI)—fields of energy around certain types of equipment that use electricity and magnets that may interfere with the normal operation of electronic devices, such as an implanted heart device. Interference occurs when the device senses energy outside the body and reacts inappropriately because it interprets the external sources as being signals from the heart.

Electrophysiologist—a cardiologist who has special training in the diagnosis and management of cardiac rhythm abnormalities.

Electrophysiology testing (EP testing)—an invasive test during which an electrophysiologist places small catheters in the heart to examine the heart's electrical system.

End of life (EOL)—a term used to indicate that the battery of an implanted heart device is depleted; at "end of life," the device automatically disables certain features in order to preserve battery strength for the most important functions.

Epicardial lead—a pacing lead attached to the outside surface (epicardium) of the heart.

Event recorder—a small ambulatory monitor that is worn for up to 4 weeks; the monitor records an EKG when activated by the patient; used as a diagnostic tool for patients who experience loss of consciousness or blackout spells or near blackout spells.

External defibrillator—emergency personnel use either manual external defibrillator equipment or a handheld automated external defibrillator (AED) to deliver defibrillation therapy shocks to treat sudden cardiac arrest or counteract atrial fibrillation or ventricular fibrillation. External defibrillators deliver therapy to the chest at very high energy levels.

Extraction—the process of removing an implanted heart device and/or leads.

H

Heart attack (myocardial infarction)—when some of the heart's blood supply is reduced or cut off, causing the heart muscle (myocardium) to die because it is deprived of its oxygen supply.

Heart block—a type of heart problem where the electrical impulses traveling from the upper chambers to the lower chambers of the heart are slowed (first degree heart block), irregularly transmitted from upper to lower chambers (second degree heart block), or completely blocked transmission between chambers (third degree heart block).

Heart failure (congestive heart failure)—a condition in which the heart can't pump enough blood to meet the needs of the body. There can be many symptoms including shortness of breath (dyspnea), fatigue, and swelling of the legs to name a few.

Holter monitor—a small ambulatory heart monitor usually worn for 24-48 hours; the monitor records an EKG and is used as a diagnostic tool for patients felt to have symptoms that could be caused by a very slow or fast heart rhythm.

Hyperarousal—physical symptoms of extreme anxiety; may include irritability, nightmares, panic attacks, and strong startle response.

I

ICD—abbreviation for "implantable cardioverter defibrillator," sometimes referred to as "defibrillator." An ICD is used to treat abnormal, fast ventricular heart rhythms.

Inappropriate shock—an ICD shock delivered for reasons other than a life-threatening arrhythmia.

Interventional cardiologist—a cardiologist with special training to treat blockage of the coronary arteries with a balloon procedure and/or stent as well as some other heart-related procedures. Interventional procedures are usually done through an artery or percutaneously as opposed to an open surgical procedure that would be performed by a cardiac surgeon.

Intrusive thoughts—repeated thoughts of a frightening event; may interfere with concentration or daily functioning.

L

Lead—a flexible wire surrounded by insulation material. The lead delivers the electrical impulse or therapy to the heart from an implanted device. It also senses the electrical activity of the heart and provides this information to the implanted device.

Left anterior descending coronary artery—one of three coronary arteries. This artery travels down the front wall of the left ventricle and often also supplies blood to the tip or apex of the left ventricle.

Left bundle branch block (LBBB)—occurs when the electrical impulse is delayed in getting through one branch, the left bundle branch, of the electrical system in the ventricles. This leads to a characteristic appearance on the EKG. It may be an indicator of a problem with the heart muscle.

Left ventricular ejection fraction (LVEF)—the percentage or fraction of blood that the left ventricle squeezes out with each beat. (See also **Ejection fraction**.) A normal LVEF is 50 to 60%.

Lower rate limit (LRL)—the slowest rate to which an implanted heart device can be set or programmed.

M

Mitral valve—one of four cardiac valves. The mitral valve is located between the upper and lower chambers on the left side of the heart.

MRI (magnetic resonance imaging)—a type of medical imaging that uses magnetic fields to create an internal view of the body. MRI can cause interference with implantable devices.

N

Neurocardiogenic syncope—a term used to describe an imbalance of the two sets of nerves that help control heart rate and blood pressure. It can result in a sudden drop in heart rate and/or blood pressure and could lead to blackout spells or near blackout spells.

P

Pacemaker—an implanted medical device that stimulates the heart muscle with timed pulses of electricity. These very small amounts of electricity cause the heart to contract, mimicking a naturally occurring heart rhythm.

Pacing, pacing therapy—a type of therapy provided by an implanted heart device to treat an abnormal heart rhythm.

Pacing threshold—a measurement of the amount of energy required to consistently capture or stimulate the heart.

Perforation—puncturing of the heart wall; a possible complication of lead placement.

Pericarditis—irritation of the sac surrounding the heart (**Pericardium**) that can be caused by a perforation.

Pericardium—the sac surrounding the heart.

Phantom shock—a phenomenon that occurs when an ICD patient believes he or she has been shocked, but when the device is interrogated there is no evidence of a shock having occurred.

Pneumothorax—a collapsed lung or portion of a lung.

Post-traumatic stress disorder (PTSD)—a collection of symptoms that may occur after a traumatic experience (see also **Avoidance behaviors, Hyperarousal, Instrusive thoughts**).

Pre-syncope—a feeling that loss of consciousness may occur—that is, a near blackout.

Primary prevention patient—a patient who has not experienced a symptomatic fast heart rhythm or sudden death but because of identified risk factors meets justification to have an ICD implanted.

Programmer—a portable desktop computer with a communication wand attached; used to interrogate and program implanted heart devices.

Pulmonic valve—one of four cardiac valves. This valve is located on the right side of the heart between the heart and vessels leading into the lungs.

Pulse generator—common term for a pacemaker, ICD, or CRT device. Refers simply to the "can."

R

Right bundle branch block (RBBB)—occurs when the electrical impulse is delayed in getting through a single electrical branch: the right bundle branch of the electrical system in the ventricles. RBBB is not usually associated with any specific heart problem and does not usually require any treatment.

Right coronary artery—one of three coronary arteries. This artery supplies blood to the back or inferior wall of the left ventricle.

S

Secondary prevention patient—a patient who meets indication for an ICD because of at least one prior symptomatic episode of a fast heart rhythm from the lower chamber of the heart.

Sensing—refers to the implanted device's ability to recognize a natural heartbeat. This is important to prevent the implanted device from competing with the patient's natural or native heart rhythm.

Septum—the muscled wall dividing the right and left sides of the heart.

Shock plan—a step-by-step plan for dealing with an ICD shock; forming a shock plan may help alleviate anxiety associated with a potential shock experience.

Single-chamber pacemaker—a pacemaker that uses one lead to stimulate a single chamber. Most commonly, this would be a lead placed in the right ventricle (also called a VVI or VVIR pacemaker) but could also be a single-chamber atrial pacemaker—that is, AAI or AAIR pacemaker.

Sinoatrial (SA) node—the heart's natural pacemaker, located in the top chamber on the right side of the heart—that is, the right atrium. Electrical impulses originate here and travel through the heart. Also called the sinus node.

Sinus bradycardia—occurs when the regular heart rate determined by the sinus node is slower than normal; in adults, a heart rate slower than 60 beats per minute is considered sinus bradycardia by definition but many adults, especially men and well-trained individuals or athletes, may have resting heart rates slower than 60 beats per minute.

Sinus node disease; sinus node dysfunction—abnormalities of the sinoatrial node (sinus node) that results in failure to provide regular electrical activation of the top chambers of the heart. This may cause intermittently slow and/or fast heart rates, or permanently slow heart rates. If symptomatic, it may require a pacemaker and/or other treatments. Sinus node dysfunction is also called sick sinus syndrome.

If the patient experiences both slow and fast heart rhythms, it is called bradycardia-tachycardia syndrome, or tachy-brady syndrome.

Sinus tachycardia—occurs when the heart rate as determined by the sinus node is faster than normal. By definition, a tachycardia is a rate greater than 100 beats per minute when at rest.

6-minute walk test—a test to assess a patient's stamina. The patient is asked to walk as far as possible within 6 minutes while the distance is measured, noting any symptoms that occur during the walk.

Sudden cardiac arrest (SCA)—also called "cardiac arrest." Failure of the heart to beat in an effective way that compromises blood flow to the body. It may be caused by the heartbeat stopping or by a very fast heart rhythm, ventricular tachycardia or fibrillation, that leads to collapse. If left untreated, it will lead to death within minutes.

Syncope—fainting, loss of consciousness, or dizziness that may be due to a transient disturbance of cardiac rhythm (arrhythmia) or other causes.

T

Tachyarrhythmia—a fast heart rhythm that may or may not also be irregular. See also **Tachycardia**.

Tachycardia—a fast heart rhythm, usually defined as greater than 100 beats per minute at rest. See also **Tachyarrhythmia**.

Tachycardia-bradycardia syndrome (Tachy/brady syndrome)—See **Sinus node dysfunction**.

Tilt-table study—performed as a diagnostic study for the diagnosis of vasovagal syncope or neurocardiogenic syncope; heart rate and blood pressure are monitored while the patient is taken from a supine position, laying down, to an almost upright position on an adjustable table and kept in that unnatural position for some length of time. Also referred to as a "head-up tilt study."

Transvenous lead—a pacing lead threaded through a vein and placed inside the heart. See also **Lead**.

Tricuspid valve—one of four heart valves. This valve is located on the right side of the heart between the upper and lower chambers.

U

Unipolar lead—a type of lead used with an implantable heart device that consists of one conductor wire surrounded by insulation.

Upper rate limit (URL)—the fastest rate that an implanted heart device can be programmed to pace the heart.

V

Vasovagal syncope—occurs when a sudden drop in heart rate and blood pressure causes dizziness, light-headedness or loss of consciousness; due to an imbalance of the nerves that help control heart rate and blood pressure; see also **Neurocardiogenic syncope**.

Ventricle, ventricles—the two lower chambers of the heart. These are called the right and left ventricles.

Ventricular fibrillation (VF)—a very fast, chaotic heart rhythm that starts in the ventricles. During VF, the heart quivers instead of contracting. If left untreated, VF is fatal.

Ventricular tachyarrhythmia— abnormally fast heart rhythms that start in the ventricles. Ventricular fibrillation (VF) and ventricular tachycardia (VT) are ventricular tachyarrhythmias.

Ventricular tachycardia (VT)—a rapid but organized heart rhythm that starts in the ventricles. During VT, the heart does not have time to fill with enough blood between heartbeats to supply the entire body with sufficient blood. VT may cause dizziness, light-headedness or complete loss of consciousness.

Index

Note: An *f* after a page number indicates a figure on that page.

A

AAI pacing mode, 20, 139
AAIR pacing mode, 20, 139
abbreviations for devices, 137
ablation equipment, interference with
    device function, 58
ablation procedures, 37, 104
active fixation, of lead, 19, 78
adjustment difficulties
    body image, 112–14
    lifestyle changes, 110–11
    trust in device, 111–12
    young patients, 114–15
advance directive, 131, 132
advisories, device, 123–27
airport metal detectors, 57
Alzheimer's disease, 132
anesthesia
    complications, 83
    implant surgery, 39, 41–42, 48, 51
    topical, 48
antiarrhythmics, 103, 141
antitachycardia pacing (ATP), 21, 89,
    103–4, 141
anti-theft devices, 57
anxiety, 105, 106–8, 110, 116–17
aorta, 2, 4
aortic valve, 2
arc welders, use after implant, 57
arm motion, after device implant, 43,
    53–54
aspirin, 39
ATP (antitachycardia pacing), 21, 89,
    103–4, 141
atrial fibrillation (AF)
    definition, 141
    description, 8–9*f*

pacemaker not used for, 17
    treatment, 37, 90
atrial flutter, 9–10*f*, 141
atrial tachyarrhythmias, 141
atrial tachycardia, 87
atrioventricular node (AV node), 6*f*, 14, 141
atrium/atria, 1, 6, 141
AV node ablation, 37
avoidance behaviors, 116, 117, 141

B

battery
    elective replacement indicator, 71,
        73, 143
    home monitoring, 74
    lifespan, 18–19, 70, 71–72
    location, 19, 72
    pacemaker, 18–19
    preserving strength of, 72
    replacement, 19, 72
    testing, 71–73
battery change, 54
beeping device, 73
bipolar lead, 20, 141
biventricular (Bi-V) devices, 23–24. *See
    also* cardiac resynchronization therapy
    (CRT) device
blood pressure, 31–32, 34, 41, 48
blood supply to heart, problems with,
    13–14. *See also* congestive heart failure;
    heart attack; heart failure
blood thinners, 38–39
body image, 112–14
    personal story, 113–14
bradycardia, 7, 37, 142
bypass surgery, 5, 142

C

can. *See* pulse generator
cardiac ablation, 37, 142
cardiac blood flow, basic concepts, 1–5, 2*f*
cardiac resynchronization therapy (CRT)
    device, 23–25. *See also* biventricular
    (Bi-V) devices
        advanced features, 73
        definition, 142
        dual-chamber, 25
        home monitoring, 74
        ICD incorporated in, 25
        leads, 24*f*, 25*f*, 49, 50
        pacing only ability, 25
        questions to ask before procedure, 36
        reasons to use, 14, 24
        single-chamber, 25
        testing prior to receiving, 34
        turning off, 130
cardiologist, 28
cardioversion, 58, 142
caregiver, types of, 7
caregiver role, 120–22
catheters, 33, 48
cell phones, 57
chainsaws, 43, 57
chambers, heart, 1. *See also* atrium/atria;
    ventricle(s)
chest tube, 80
CHF. *See* congestive heart failure (CHF)
children
        extraction of device, 91
        heart rates in, 8
        pacemaker for, 17*f*
chiropractic equipment, interference with
    device function, 58
cholesterol level, 34
circumflex coronary artery, 4, 5, 142
clinical depression, 109
clopidogrel (Plavix), 39
collapsed lung (pneumothorax), 79–80
communication wand, 66, 74
communicator, 74–75
complications
        directly related to implant
            procedure, 77–83
        anesthesia, 83
        collapsed lung, 79–80
        infection, 80–82

lead dislodgement, 78–79
        perforation of heart wall, 82
        extraction procedures, 92
        heart attack, 83–84
        later complications, 84–87
        erosion, 86–87*f*
        pain, 85–86
        unacceptable function of lead, 84–85
        risk of death, 83
        unique to ICDs, 87–92
        extractions, 91–92
        inappropriate shocks, 87–89
        multiple shocks, 89–90
        therapies accidentally turned off,
            90–91
conduction pathways, 6*f*
congestive heart failure (CHF), 14, 34. *See
    also* cardiac resynchronization therapy
    (CRT) device; heart failure; implantable
    cardioverter defibrillator (ICD)
consciousness, loss of, 22, 60, 62, 118–19
coping matters, 106–10. *See also*
    adjustment difficulties
        anxiety symptoms, 106–8
        depression symptoms, 108–10
coronary arteries, 4*f*–5*f*, 13
Coumadin (warfarin), 38
CRT. *See* cardiac resynchronization therapy
    (CRT) device
CRT-D, 25, 137
CRT-P, 25, 137

D

dabigatran (Pradaxa), 39
DDD pacing mode, 20, 139
DDDR pacing mode, 20, 139
death. *See also* end-of-life decisions
        risk during extraction, 92
        risk during implantation, 83
        from third degree heart block, 12
        from ventricular fibrillation, 22
defibrillation, 142
defibrillation threshold testing (DFT), 51,
    142
defibrillator, 142. *See also* implantable
    cardioverter defibrillator (ICD)
dementia, 132
depression, 105, 108–10
device. *See also* cardiac resynchronization

therapy (CRT) device; device
manufacturer; implantable cardioverter
defibrillator (ICD); pacemaker (PM)
    abbreviations, 137
    advisories, 123–27
    as cure, 63
    how to choose, 36
    settings, 50–51, 67–68
device extraction. *See* extraction
device manufacturer
    activity questions, 44
    availability of devices, 36
    contact information, 135
    educational materials, 55
    patient ID card, 56, 63, 66
    technical questions, 63
device selection, 36
device settings, 50–51, 67–68
DFT (defibrillation threshold testing), 51,
    142
diaphragm, stimulation of, 85
diuretics/water pills, 39
DNR (do not resuscitate) order, 131
doctor
    choosing prior to receiving device,
        28, 35–36
    electrophysiologist, 6, 28, 33, 103,
        143
    heart failure specialist, 28, 34
    interventional cardiologist, 5, 144
    questions to ask after procedure, 63
    questions to ask before procedure,
        35–36, 37, 44
do not resuscitate (DNR) order, 131
driving restrictions, 42, 60–62
dropped/missed heart beat, 11
dual-chamber internal cardioverter
    defibrillator, 21
dual-chamber pacemaker, 20, 142
Dyazide (hydrochlorothiazide), 39

E
ECG (EKG) (electrocardiogram)
    ambulatory monitor for recording,
        29–30
    definition, 143
    event recorder for recording, 30*f*–31
    how it works, 29*f*
    to test lead dislodgement, 79
    tilt-table test and, 31–32

echocardiogram, 33–34, 143. *See also* left
    ventricular ejection fraction
edema, 14
education, patient, 15, 40–41, 52, 55, 135
ejection fraction (EF), 14, 34, 143. *See also*
    left ventricular ejection fraction (LVEF)
elective replacement indicator (ERI), 71,
    73, 143
electrical block. *See* heart block
electrical system of heart
    overview, 6*f*
    problems with, 7–13
ECG/EKG. *See* ECG (EKG)
    (electrocardiogram)
electrocautery, 58, 143
electrodes, lead, 19
electromagnetic interference (EMI), 56–58,
    143
electrophysiologist, 6, 28, 33, 103, 143
electrophysiology testing (EP testing), 33,
    143
emergencies, 44, 89, 118–19
EMI (electromagnetic interference), 56–58,
    143
end of life (EOL), of battery, 72, 143
end-of-life decisions, 127–33
    planning end-of-life care, 131–33
    request device be turned off,
        128–31
enlarged heart, 3*f*. *See also* left ventricle
epicardial lead, 143
ERI (elective replacement indicator), 71,
    73, 143
erosion, of leads or devices, 86–87*f*
event recorder, 30*f*–31, 143
external defibrillator, 93, 143
extraction
    complications, 91–92
    before cremation, 130
    definition, 82, 143

F
failure to capture, 84
fainting. *See* syncope
family and friends
    advisories, reaction to, 124–25
    anxiety among, 108
    caregiver role by, 120–22
    shock plan and, 118–19

fibrosis (scar tissue), 54, 56, 78, 79, 84, 86, 92
first degree heart block, 11
fluid, accumulation of, 14, 73
follow-up care
    advanced features of device, 73
    beeping device, 73
    device settings, 67–68
    device testing, 68–73
    home monitoring system, 74–76
    how device is checked, 66
    importance of, 127
    schedule for, 65–66
frozen shoulder, 54
furosemide (Lasix), 39

G
gender, differences in heart rate, 8
general anesthetic, 83
glossary, 141–48
Glucophage (metformin) 40

H
head-up tilt study. *See* tilt-table study
heart
    blood supply problems, 13–14
    conduction pathways of, 6*f*
    electrical system problems, 7–13
    enlarged, 3*f*
    normal, 1*f*
heart attack (myocardial infarction)
    causes, 13
    definition, 143–44
    difference from sudden cardiac
        arrest, 13
    risk during surgery, 83–84
heart block, 10–12
    definition, 144
    first degree, 11
    left bundle, 12, 144
    right bundle, 12, 146
    second degree, 11*f*
    third degree, 11–12*f*
heart failure (congestive heart failure), 3*f*
    definition, 144
    doctor for, 28, 34
    leads for CRT device, 40, 49
    symptoms, 14
    treatment, 24–25

Heart Failure Society of America, 28
heart failure specialist, 28, 34
Heart Rhythm Society, 28
heart tracing. *See* ECG (EKG) (electrocardiogram)
heavy equipment, use after device implant, 43
Holter monitor, 29–30, 144
home monitoring systems, 74–76, 85
household appliances, use after device implant, 43–44
hunting and shooting, after device implant, 43
hydrochlorothiazide (Dyazide), 39
hyperarousal, 116, 144

I
ibuprofen, 82
ICD. *See* implantable cardioverter defibrillator (ICD)
ID card, 56, 63, 66
implantable cardiac devices. *See* cardiac resynchronization therapy (CRT) device; implantable cardioverter defibrillator (ICD); pacemaker (PM)
implantable cardioverter defibrillator (ICD), 20–23, 25
    advanced features, 73
    complications, 87–92
    components, 21
    definition, 144
    driving restrictions, 42, 60–62
    dual-chamber, 21
    electromagnetic interference, 56
    extraction, 91–92
    follow-up care, 65
    home monitoring, 74, 75
    how it works, 21–23
    leads, 22–23
    pacemaker included in, 20–21
    programming, 68
    pulse generator, 21
    questions to ask before procedure, 35–36
    reason to use, 14
    shocks (see shocks)
    single-chamber, 21
    testing during implantation, 51
    testing prior to receiving, 33–34

Index

therapies accidentally turned off,
90–91
turning off, 129–30
inappropriate shocks, 87–89, 94, 144
infants, heart rate in, 8
infection, 55, 80–82, 91
inferior vena cava, 2f
insulin, 39–40
interventional cardiologist, 5, 144
interventional procedures. See bypass
surgery
intrusive thoughts, 116, 144
iPods, 57

L

Lasix (furosemide), 39
LBBB (left bundle branch block), 12, 144
leads
bipolar, 20, 141
complications, 78–83, 84–85
conductor wire, 71
CRT, 24f, 25f, 49, 50
defibrillators, 22–23
definition, 144
diaphragm/muscle stimulation by, 85
dislodgement, 78–79f, 84
driving restrictions, 42
electrodes, 19
epicardial, 143
extraction, 91–92
impedance level testing, 71
insulation, 19–20, 71, 84–85
MRIs and, 58
pacemaker, 17, 19f–20
placement during surgery, 49–50
restrictions to protect, 43, 54
shocking coils, 23
transvenous, 147
unipolar, 20, 147
varieties, 19
left anterior descending coronary artery,
4f, 5, 144
left bundle branch, 6
left bundle branch block (LBBB), 12, 144
left main coronary artery, 4
left ventricle
blood supply to, 4–5
enlarged, 3f, 14, 24
heart attack and, 13
role of, 1–2

left ventricular ejection fraction (LVEF).
See also ejection fraction (EF)
decrease in, 14
definition, 3, 145
normal value, 3, 34
liability, 42
lidocaine, 48
lifestyle changes. See adjustment
difficulties; restrictions after implant
lightheadedness, 8, 70
lithium-iodine batteries, 18–19
lower rate limit (LRL), 67, 68, 145
lungs
collapsed, 79–80
role in blood circulation, 2
LVEF. See left ventricular ejection fraction
(LVEF)

M

magnetic resonance imaging (MRI), 58,
145
medications, and surgery, 38–40
metal detectors, airport, 57
metformin (Glucophage), 40
microwave oven use, and pacemakers, 43
missed/dropped heart beat, 11
mitral valve, 3, 145
MRI (magnetic resonance imaging), 58, 145

N

NEEDS, 131
neurocardiogenic syncope, 31, 32, 145

O

occupational restrictions, 58, 110–11
operating room. See procedure (operating)
room
oral antibiotics, 55
outpatient procedures, 52

P

pacemaker (PM), 17–20
altering settings and functions of, 19
battery, 18–19
components of, 17
definition, 145
driving restrictions, 42
dual-chamber, 20, 142
electromagnetic interference, 56

follow-up care, 65
home monitoring systems, 74
within ICD, 20–21
inhibited, 138
leads, 17f, 19f–20
microwave oven use, 43
need for, 12, 28, 37
pacing mode designations, 20,
    138–40
programming, 67–68
pulse generator, 17f, 18–19
questions to ask before procedure,
    35
rate responsive, 138–39
replacement, 19
sensing, 70
settings and functions, altering, 19
single-chamber, 20, 146
size of, 21f
temporary, 44
testing prior to receiving, 28–32
turning off, 128–29
pacemaker circuitry, 18, 19
pacing, pacing therapy, 145
pacing threshold, 69–70
paddles, 93
pain
    after generator change, 56
    after surgery, 53
    chest, 82, 118
    fear of before surgery, 41–42
    at implant site, 85–86
    from shock, 94, 95, 119
pain medication, 55, 86
passing out. See also syncope
    driving restrictions and, 59–61
passive fixation, of lead, 19, 78
patient education, 15, 40–41, 52, 55, 135
patient education websites, 135
perforation, 82, 145
pericarditis, 82, 145
pericardium, 82, 145
phantom shocks, 97–102, 145
Plavix (clopidogrel), 39
"plumbers," 5
PM. See pacemaker (PM)
pneumothorax, 79–80, 145
pocket pain, 86
polyurethane insulation for lead, 20

post-traumatic stress disorder (PTSD),
    116–17, 145
power tools, use after device implant, 43,
    57
Pradaxa (dabigatran), 39
preparation for device procedure, 38–40.
    See also procedure, after; procedure
    (operating) room
        anesthesia, 39, 41–42
        day of surgery, 40–41
        educational session, 40–41
        medications, 38–40
        night before surgery, 38
        before procedure, 41
        during procedure, 41–42
        restrictions after implant, 42–44
pre-syncope, 28, 145
primary prevention patient, 33, 145
procedure, after. See also preparation
    for device procedure; procedure
    (operating) room
        driving, 42, 59–61
        educational materials, 55
        electromagnetic interferences, do's
            and don'ts, 56–58
        incision care, 55
        restrictions after implant, 42–44
        resumption of usual activities, 58–59
        soreness after surgery, 53
procedure (operating) room. See also
    preparation for device procedure;
    procedure, after
        actual procedure, 47–52
        anesthesia, 48
        device placement, 48–49, 50
        feeling of coldness, 45
        lead placement, 49–50
        length of procedure, 52
        "making the pocket," 49
        preoperative preparations, 45–47
        prepping upper chest, 47
        safeguards, 46–47
programmer, 19, 50–51, 66, 79, 145
pulmonary arteries, 2f
pulmonary veins, 2f
pulmonic valve, 2, 146
pulse generator
    battery, 18–19, 72
    changing, 54, 55–56

definition, 146
internal cardioverter defibrillator, 21
pacemaker, 17*f*, 18–19
pacemaker circuitry, 18, 19
parts of, 18
programmer, communication with, 19

Q
questions
about extractions, 91
to ask after procedure, 63
to ask before procedure, 35–36, 37, 44
reasons to ask, 15
technical, 63

R
radiation treatment, interference with device function, 58
rapid pacing therapy, 68, 89, 133
rate responsive pacemakers, 139
RBBB (right bundle branch block), 12, 146
recalls (device advisories), 124–27
recovery room, 52
red blood cells, 2
restrictions after implant, 42–44
arm motion on implant side, 43, 53–54
driving, 42, 59–62
household appliances, 43–44
hunting or shooting, 43
occupations, 58, 110–11
power tool or heavy equipment use, 43, 57
resumption of usual activities, 58–59
right atrium, 2
right bundle branch, 6
right bundle branch block (RBBB), 12, 146
right coronary artery, 4*f*, 146
right ventricle, 2

S
safety margin, pacing, 70
SCA. *See* sudden cardiac arrest
scar tissue (fibrosis), 54, 56, 78, 79, 84, 86, 92
screw mechanism, for lead, 19, 49–50, 78
secondary prevention patient, 33, 146

second degree heart block, 11*f*
second opinion, 34
sensing, 70–71, 146
sensitivity level, 70–71
septum, 146
settings, device, 50–51, 67–68
shocking coils, 23
shock plan, 99, 117–20, 146
shocks
coping with, 115–17
description, 95–96
electromagnetic interference, 56
home monitoring, 75
inappropriate, 87–89, 94, 144
multiple, 89–90
pain from, 94, 95, 119
personal story, 96–97, 100–102
phantom, 97–102, 145
planning for, 99, 117–20
prevention, 102–4
ATP, 103–4
medication, 103
VT ablation, 104
state of mind and, 96–102
threshold testing during implantation, 51
what shocks feel like, 94
shortness of breath, 14, 118. *See also* heart failure
sick sinus syndrome. *See* sinus node dysfunction
silicone rubber insulation for lead, 20
single-chamber ICD, 21
single-chamber pacemaker, 20, 146
sinoatrial (SA) node, 146
sinus bradycardia, 8, 146
sinus node, 6*f*, 14. *See also* sinoatrial (SA) node
sinus node disease, 7, 146–47
sinus node dysfunction, 7*f*, 14
sinus tachycardia, 8, 87, 147
6-minute walk test, 34–35, 147
slow heart rate, preventing. *See* pacemaker
spouses, of ICD patients, 120–22
personal story, 121
stents, 5
stroke, risk during surgery, 83
sudden cardiac arrest (SCA)
causes, 14

definition, 147

difference from heart attack, 13

superior vena cava, 2*f*

support groups, 99

surgery. *See* preparation for device procedure

syncope

definition, 28, 147

neurocardiogenic, 31, 32, 145

vasovagal, 31, 32, 147

T

tachyarrhythmia

atrial, 141

definition, 147

treatment, 20

tachycardia, 7, 20, 147

tachycardia-bradycardia syndrome (tachy/ brady syndrome), 7*f*, 147. *See also* Sinus node dysfunction

temporary pacemaker, 44

test/testing

after implantation, 68–69, 79

battery, 71–73

defibrillation threshold, 51, 142

impedance, 71

lead dislodgement, 79, 84

lead impedance level, 71

pacing threshold, 69–70

prior to receiving device, 28–34

sensing, 70–71

6-minute walk test, 34–35, 147

tilt-table test, 31–32*f*, 147

third degree heart block, 11–12*f*

tilt-table study, 31–32*f*, 147

titanium, 18

topical anesthetic, 48

trans-telephonic monitoring, 74

transvenous lead, 147

traveling, after device implant, 63

tricuspid valve, 2, 147

trusting your device, 111–12

U

ultrasonic transducer, 33

ultrasound. *See* echocardiogram

unipolar lead, 20, 147

upper rate limit (URL), 66–67, 147

V

vasovagal syncope, 31, 32, 147. *See also* neurocardiogenic syncope

veins, role in circulation, 2*f*

vena cava, 2*f*

ventricle(s)

definition, 148

left (see left ventricle)

right, 2

ventricular fibrillation (VF)

causes, 14

definition, 148

treatment, 22–23*f*, 87, 88, 95, 103

ventricular tachyarrhythmia, 148

ventricular tachycardia (VT)

causes, 14

definition, 148

treatment, 21, 22*f*, 23, 37, 87, 88, 95, 103, 104

VT ablation, 104

VVI pacing mode, 20, 139–40

VVIR pacing mode, 20, 139

W

warfarin (Coumadin), 38

water pills, 39

welding equipment, 43, 57

wires. *See* leads

wound check, 55

X

x-rays

to guide lead placement, 49

to test lead dislodgement, 79, 84

Y

young patients, 114–15. *See also* children